Affiliated with Molecular Biology of Hematopoiesis Symposium

Acta Hæmatologica

Founded 1948 by E. Meulengracht, K. Rohr, and G. Rosenow
Continued by H. Lüdin (1960–1977), U. Bucher (1977–1983), R.S. Hillman (1978–1987), H.R. Marti (1983–1988), E.A. Beck (1984–1988), B. Ramot (1989–1995)

KARGER

Printed in Switzerland on acid-free paper by Reinhardt Druck, Basel

Appears 6-weekly: 2 volumes per year (8 issues)

Guidelines for Authors

Acta Haematologica

Submission

Only original papers written in English are considered and should be sent to:

Prof. I. Ben-Bassat
S. Karger AG
Editorial Office Acta Haematologica
P.O. Box
CH–4009 Basel (Switzerland)
Tel. +41 61 306 1358
Fax +41 61 306 1434
E-Mail b.brogli@karger.ch

Mailing address for courier deliveries only:

Allschwilerstr. 10
CH–4055 Basel (Switzerland)

Manuscripts should be submitted in triplicate (with three sets of illustrations of which one is an original), typewritten double-spaced on one side of the paper, with a wide margin.

Conditions

All manuscripts are subject to editorial review. Manuscripts are received with the explicit understanding that they are not under simultaneous consideration by any other publication. Submission of an article for publication implies the transfer of the copyright from the author to the publisher upon acceptance. Accepted papers become the permanent property of 'Acta Haematologica' and may not be reproduced by any means, in whole or in part, without the written consent of the publisher. It is the author's responsibility to obtain permission to reproduce illustrations, tables, etc. from other publications.

Arrangement

Recommendation for Usage of Units and Abbreviations: The Editorial Board of 'Acta Haematologica' supports the recommendations of the 'International Committee for Standardization in Hematology' for using the SI (Système International d'Unités) equivalents in haematological literature. The standard abbreviations used for measurements of weight, length, volume, and time (i.e. mg, cm, ml, min) are used without definition. The abbreviations listed on the opposite page also require no definition. Please note that punctuation is not needed. When using other abbreviations, spell out the name in full at the first mention, and follow with the abbreviation in parentheses.

Title page: The first page of each paper should indicate the title, the authors' names, and the institute where the work was conducted. A short title for use as running head as well as the full address of the author to whom correspondence should be sent are also required.

Full address: The exact postal address complete with postal code must be given at the bottom of the title page. Please also supply phone and fax numbers, as well as your e-mail address.

Key words: For indexing purposes, a list of 3–10 key words in English is essential.

Abstract: Each paper needs an abstract of up to 10 lines.

Small type: Paragraphs which can or must be set in smaller type (case histories, test methods, etc.) should be indicated with a 'p' (petit) in the margin on the left-hand side.

Footnotes: Avoid footnotes. When essential, they are numbered consecutively and typed at the foot of the appropriate page.

Tables and illustrations: Tables and illustrations (both numbered in Arabic numerals) should be prepared on separate sheets. Tables require a heading and figures a legend, also prepared on a separate sheet. For the reproduction of illustrations, only good drawings and original photographs can be accepted; negatives or photocopies cannot be used. Due to technical reasons, figures with a screen background should not be submitted. When possible, group several illustrations on one block for reproduction (max. size 180 × 223 mm) or provide crop marks. On the back of each illustration, indicate its number, the author's name, and 'top' with a soft pencil.

Color illustrations: Up to 6 color illustrations per page can be integrated within the text at the reduced price of CHF 660.–/USD 545.00 per page. Color illustrations are reproduced at the author's expense.

References: In the text identify references by Arabic numerals [in square brackets]. Material submitted for publication but not yet accepted should be noted as 'unpublished data' and not be included in the reference list. The list of references should include only those publications which are cited in the text. Do not alphabetize; number references in the order in which they are first mentioned in the text. The surnames of the authors followed by initials should be given. There should be no punctuation other than a comma to separate the authors. Cite all authors, 'et al' is not sufficient. Abbreviate journal names according to the Index Medicus system. (Also see International Committee of Medical Journal Editors: Uniform requirements for manuscripts submitted to biomedical journals. N Engl J Med 1997;336:309–315.)

Examples
(a) *Papers published in periodicals:* Sun J, Koto H, Chung KF: Interaction of ozone and allergen challenges on bronchial responsiveness and inflammation in sensitised guinea pigs. Int Arch Allergy Immunol 1997;112:191–195.
(b) *Monographs:* Matthews DE, Farewell VT: Using and Understanding Medical Statistics, ed 3, revised. Basel, Karger, 1996.
(c) *Edited books:* Parren PWHI, Burton DR: Antibodies against HIV-1 from phage display libraries: Mapping of an immune response and progress towards antiviral immunotherapy; in Capra JD (ed): Antibody Engineering. Chem Immunol. Basel, Karger, 1997, vol 65, pp 18–56.

Page Charges

Authors are charged CHF 138.–/USD 98.00 per printed page for the first 6 pages and CHF 275.–/USD 196.00 for each additional page, including tables, illustrations, and references. 1 printed page is equal to approximately 3 manuscript pages.

Rapid Communication

Manuscripts intended for rapid communication must present new findings of sufficient importance to justify their accelerated acceptance. They should follow the general arrangement of research papers except that the separate sections should not be formally titled. They should not be more than three pages in length (including figures, tables and references). Proofs are checked by the Main Editor and not sent to the authors. Review will be rapid, and once accepted, the paper will be included in the next planned issue. If manuscripts require significant change after editing they will be treated as brief communications and returned to the authors for correction.

Brief Communication

The general arrangement for brief communications is the same as for research papers except that the manuscript is not divided into separate sections formally entitled introduction, methods, results, discussion. No abstract is required. These should not be more than 3 pages in length.

Letter to the Editor

Comments and responses to previously published articles and other short correspondences are welcome. They should be limited to 1 or 1 1/2 manuscript pages with a general arrangement as specified for Brief Communications.

Galley Proofs

Unless indicated otherwise, galley proofs are sent to the first-named author and should be returned with the least possible delay. Alterations made in galley proofs, other than the correction of printer's errors, are charged to the author. No page proofs are supplied.

Reprints

Order forms and a price list are sent with the galley proofs. Orders submitted after the issue is printed are subject to considerably higher prices.

KARGER

Fax +41 61 306 12 34
E-Mail karger@karger.ch
www.karger.com

The Guidelines for Authors are available at:
www.karger.com/journals/aha/aha_gl.htm

General Information

Acta Hæmatologica

Publication data: 'Acta Haematologica' is published 8 times a year. Volumes 107, 108 with 4 issues each appear in 2002.

Subscription rates: Subscriptions run for a full calendar year. Prices are given per volume.

Personal subscription:

Subscription + postage and handling
CHF 322.– + CHF 19.20 Europe
CHF 322.– + CHF 28.50 Overseas
USD 247.50 + USD 19.20
+ online subscription per volume:
CHF 39.– / USD 30.00
(Must be in the name of, billed to, and paid by an individual. Order must be marked 'personal subscription'.)

Institutional subscription:

Subscription + postage and handling
CHF 644.– + CHF 24.– Europe
CHF 644.– + CHF 35.60 Overseas
USD 495.00 + USD 24.
+ online subscription per volume:
CHF 58.– / USD 45.00

Airmail postage: CHF 24.–, USD 20.00.
(Extra per volume.)

Discount subscription prices:
International Society of Haematology

Microforms: Please direct all enquiries and orders to: University Microfilms Inc.
300 North Zeeb Road, P.O. Box 1346
Ann Arbor, MI 48106-1346 (USA)

Subscription orders: Orders can be placed at agencies, bookstores, directly with the Publisher
S. Karger AG, P.O. Box,
CH–4009 Basel (Switzerland)
or with any of the following distributors:

Deutschland: S. Karger GmbH, Postfach
D–79095 Freiburg

France: Librairie Luginbühl
36, bd de Latour-Maubourg, F–75007 Paris

Great Britain, Ireland: S. Karger Publishers
58 Grove Hill Road
Tunbridge Wells, Kent TN1 1SP, UK

USA: S. Karger Publishers, Inc.
26 West Avon Road, P.O. Box 529
Farmington, CT 06085, USA

India, Bangladesh, Sri Lanka:
Panther Publishers Private Ltd.
39, 6th Cross
Wilson Gardens
Bangalore 560 027, India

Japan: Katakura Libri, Inc.
2F, Marushima Bldg, 4-6-17, Yushima,
Bunkyo-ku, Tokyo 113-0034, Japan

Change of address: Both old and new address should be sent to the subscription source.

Single issues and back volumes: Information can be obtained through the Publisher.

Advertising: Correspondence and rate requests should be addressed to the Publisher.

Bibliographic indices: This journal is regularly listed in bibliographic services, including *Current Contents®*.

Book Reviews: Books are accepted for review by special agreement.

Copying: This journal has been registered with the Copyright Clearance Center (CCC), as indicated by the code appearing on the first page of each article.
For readers in the US, this code signals consent for copying of articles for personal or internal use, or for the personal or internal use of specific clients, provided that the stated fee is paid per copy directly to
Copyright Clearance Center Inc.
222 Rosewood Drive
Danvers, MA 01923 (USA)
A copy of the first page of the article must accompany payment. Consent does not extend to copying for general distribution, for promotion, for creating new works, or for resale. In these cases, specific written permission must be obtained from the copyright owner,
S. Karger AG,
P.O. Box, CH–4009 Basel (Switzerland).

Usage of Units and Abbreviations

Entity	Abbreviation	Recommended SI equivalent	Not recommended
Red blood cell count	RBC	10^{12}/l	10^6/mm^3
White blood cell count	WBC	10^9/l	10^3/mm^3
Platelet count		... × 10^9/l	... × 10^3/mm^3
Reticulocyte count		% (or ... × 10^9/l)	% (or ../mm^3)
Haemoglobin	Hb	g/dl[a]	g/100 ml
Packed cell volume	PCV	ratio[b]	%
Mean cell volume	MCV	fl	
Mean cell haemoglobin	MCH	pg	
Mean cell haemoglobin concentration	MCHC	g/dl	%
Mean cell diameter	MCD	μm	
Sedimentation rate	ESR	mm in 1 h[c]	
Plasma haemoglobin	Plasma Hb	mg/l	mg/100 ml
Serum vitamin B_{12}		ng/l	
Serum folate		μg/l	
Serum iron		μmol/l	μg/100 ml
Total iron binding capacity	TIBC	μmol/l	μg/100 ml
Unsaturated iron binding capacity	UIBC	μmol/l	μg/100 ml
Transferrin		g/l	mg/100 ml
Serum haptoglobin		g/l	mg/100 ml
Plasma fibrinogen		g/l	mg/100 ml

a The concentration for Hb only is expressed as ../dl and not ../l or ../100 ml.
b No unit necessary, 1/1 is implied.
c Indicate method only if other than Westergren.

KARGER

Fax +41 61 306 12 34
E-Mail karger@karger.ch
www.karger.com

The Journal Home Page is available at:
www.karger.com/journals/aha

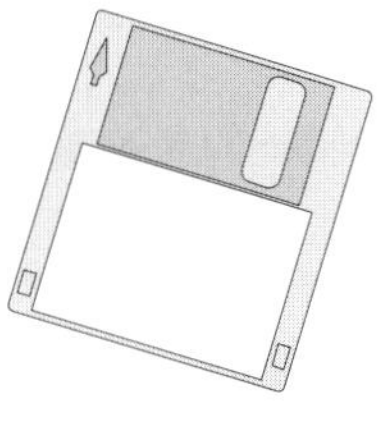

Disk Submission

A **comprehensive version** of these guidelines for the **submission of manuscripts and illustrations on disk** can be accessed online under **www.karger.com/journals/disksub.htm** or requested as a leaflet from the editorial department.

Please follow the general rules on style and arrangement in the **'Guidelines for Authors'** of the journal. Submit a **double-spaced printout** of your manuscript matching the file on disk exactly.

Technical Information
Store only data pertinent to this manuscript. Include your fonts (screen and printer fonts for Macintosh). For a **text only** manuscript, use a 3.5-inch disk. For **text and illustrations,** use 3.5 or 5.25 Magneto Optical Disc; CD-ROM (DOS or hybrid); iomage Zip/DOS (100 MB), or 44 MB, 88 MB or 200 MB SyQuest. Compress extensive data using ZIP format.

Data Description
Label your disk with the **title of the journal or book** for which it is submitted; a **short version** of the paper's title; your **name,** postal and e-mail address, fax and phone number; **hard- and software** used, including the version; and the **complete list of the file names.** File names consist of eight characters before the dot identifying the file and three characters after the dot identifying the application.

Text and Format
The **preferred word-processing package is MS-Word.** Other commonly used PC text programs and ASCII formats are accepted.
Update your data when you revise subsequent to the reviewer's or editor's decision and mark revisions clearly. Manuscripts accepted for publication are subject to **copy editing:** changes and/or questions will be marked in the manuscript, which will be returned to you with your disk and the galley proofs for checking.
Enter your text continuously flush left. Do not use any layout functions. Do not split words at the end of a line. **Do not use indentations.** Use a blank line before and a hard return at the end of paragraphs.
Arrange headings flush left. Insert only **one space after punctuation marks.** Insert Greek letters, mathematical symbols etc. with your word-processing program. Use **boldface and italics** as well as sub- and superscript where appropriate.
Tables are part of the text and should be placed at the end of the text file. Separate the individual parts of a table by lines. Use the tabulator instead of spaces. Format operation data on one line in the same column. **Legends to illustrations are part of the text** and should also be listed at the end of the text file.

Illustrations
Store illustrations as separate files: do not integrate them in your text. Export **line drawings/vector graphics** as TIF, EPS or WMF format. Use Photoshop for processing and retouching **scanned halftone images.** Save the original scan and the processed version. Export **black and white or color images** as TIF or EPS format in their anticipated size in print.
For detailed information on how to submit illustration data on disk please consult the leaflet or **www.karger.com/journals/disksub.htm.**

KI 98 DISK

KARGER

Fax + 41 61 306 12 34
E-Mail karger@karger.ch
www.karger.com

The Journal Home Page is available at:
www.karger.com/journals/aha

Acta
Hæmatologica

Angiogenesis in Hematology

Editors
Rosario Giustolisi, Catania
Francesco Di Raimondo, Catania

15 figures and 11 tables, 2001

KARGER

Basel · Freiburg · Paris · London · New York ·
New Delhi · Bangkok · Singapore · Tokyo · Sydney

S. Karger
Medical and Scientific Publishers
Basel · Freiburg · Paris · London
New York · New Delhi · Bangkok
Singapore · Tokyo · Sydney

Drug Dosage
The authors and the publisher have exerted every effort to ensure that drug selection and dosage set forth in this text are in accord with current recommendations and practice at the time of publication. However, in view of ongoing research, changes in government regulations, and the constant flow of information relating to drug therapy and drug reactions, the reader is urged to check the package insert for each drug for any change in indications and dosage and for added warnings and precautions. This is particularly important when the recommended agent is a new and/or infrequently employed drug.

P.O. Box, CH–4009 Basel (Switzerland)
Printed in Switzerland on acid-free paper by
Reinhardt Druck, Basel
ISBN 3–8055–7320–0

KARGER

Fax + 41 61 306 12 34
E-Mail karger@karger.ch
www.karger.com

Vol. 106, No. 4, 2001

Acta Hæmatologica

Contents

KARGER

Fax + 41 61 306 12 34
E-Mail karger@karger.ch
www.karger.com

Access to full text and tables of contents,
including tentative ones for forthcoming issues:
www.karger.com/journals/aha/aha_bk.htm

Acta Haematologica

Acta Haematol 2001;106:147

Foreword

The interest in studying angiogenesis has started in oncology and later spread to other fields of medicine, including hematology. While in oncology most studies are directed toward a better definition of the prognostic significance of angiogenic phenomena in cancer patients, among hematologists there is a strong interest in the involvement of angiogenesis not only in malignant diseases but also in the development and regulation of normal hematopoiesis. In this light there are many novel and interesting reports indicating that, in normal ontogeny, hematopoiesis is associated with angiogenesis and this finding has led to a reappraisal of a very old concept: the presence of a common progenitor, called hemangioblast, that gives rise to both the endothelial and hematopoietic lineages. This concept was first formulated almost one century ago but it could not be confirmed for a long time. Studies on angiogenesis have the merit not only of having taken up this old idea but also, as a consequence, of having provided new perspectives on the concept of a wide plasticity of stem cells. These studies are also of clinical utility because they can provide new insights into the pathophysiology of hematological malignancies and give some evidence that angiogenesis is critical for the development of numerous different hematological diseases. This implies that an antiangiogenic strategy may be of value in diseases such as acute and chronic leukemias, lymphomas and multiple myeloma. The biology of angiogenesis and its relationship with hematopoiesis are discussed in the first part of this supplement to *Acta Haematologica* while studies dealing with the importance of angiogenesis and antiangiogenic drugs in these diseases are addressed in the second part. The last chapter discusses the role of angiogenesis in a unique hematological disorder such as the Rendu-Osler disease.

The large amount of information that we see every day published in the international literature can be somehow confounding. We hope that this supplement will give some basic and up-to-date information that can help define the state of art of hematological research in the field of angiogenesis.

Finally, we wish to thank the authors for their contribution and S. Karger AG for publishing this supplement.

Rosario Giustolisi
Francesco Di Raimondo

KARGER

Fax + 41 61 306 12 34
E-Mail karger@karger.ch
www.karger.com

0001–5792/01/1064–0147$17.50/0

Accessible online at:
www.karger.com/journals/aha

Acta Hæmatologica

Acta Haematol 2001;106:148–156

The Role of Vascular Endothelial Growth Factor in Angiogenesis

Napoleone Ferrara Hans-Peter Gerber

Department of Molecular Oncology, Genentech, Inc., South San Francisco, Calif., USA

Key Words

Angiogenesis · Apoptosis · Endothelium · Retinopathy · Tumor growth · Tyrosine kinases · Vascular endothelial growth factor

Abstract

Vascular endothelial growth factor (VEGF) is an endothelial cell-specific mitogen and an angiogenic inducer as well as a mediator of vascular permeability. The biological effects of VEGF are mediated by two tyrosine kinase receptors, Flt-1 (VEGFr-1) and KDR (VEGFR-2). VEGF is essential for developmental angiogenesis and is also required for female reproductive functions and endochondral bone formation. Substantial evidence also implicates VEGF in tumors and intraocular neovascular syndromes. Currently, several clinical trials are ongoing to test the hypothesis that inhibition of VEGF activity may be beneficial for these conditions.

Introduction

Over the last decade, extensive work has been done on members of the vascular endothelial growth factor (VEGF) gene family. There is strong evidence that this family plays a fundamental role in the growth and differentiation of vascular as well as lymphatic endothelial cells. This family comprises several members including VEGF, placenta growth factor, VEGF-B, VEGF-C, VEGF-D and two VEGF-like proteins encoded by two strains of the parapoxvirus *orf* virus [1–3]. In particular, VEGF [4], referred to also as VEGF-A, is a major regulator of normal and abnormal angiogenesis, including that associated with tumors and several intraocular syndromes [5–7]. VEGF inhibitors are being currently tested in numerous clinical trials [8].

Biological Actions of VEGF

VEGF was characterized as a mitogen for vascular endothelial cells derived from arteries, veins and lymphatics [1, 9–11]. However, recent studies have reported mitogenic effects of VEGF also on a few nonendothelial cell types [12–14]. There is strong evidence that VEGF is a key survival factor for endothelial cells, both in vitro and in vivo [15–19]. Consistent with a prosurvival activity, VEGF induces expression of the antiapoptotic proteins Bcl-2 and A1 in human endothelial cells [16]. There is clear evidence that the survival activity is mediated by the PI 3′ kinase/Akt pathway [17]. Recent studies have shown that VE-cadherin is required for the transmission of the VEGF endothelial survival signal to Akt and Bcl-2, via complex formation with KDR, beta-catenin, and PI 3′ kinase [20].

KARGER

Fax + 41 61 306 12 34
E-Mail karger@karger.ch
www.karger.com

0001–5792/01/1064–0148$17.50/0

Accessible online at:
www.karger.com/journals/aha

Napoleone Ferrara
Department of Molecular Oncology, Genentech, Inc.
1 DNA Way
South San Francisco, CA 94080 (USA)
Tel. +1 650 225 2968, Fax +1 650 225 6327, E-Mail nf@gene.com

VEGF is known also as vascular permeability factor based on its ability to induce vascular leakage in the guinea pig skin [21, 22]. Dvorak [23] proposed that an increase in microvascular permeability to proteins is a crucial step in angiogenesis. According to this hypothesis, induced leakage of plasma proteins and formation of an extravascular fibrin gel would be sufficient for endothelial cell growth; the role of mitogenic growth factors would be to augment this process [24]. Therefore, a major role in angiogenesis for a molecule-like VEGF would be enhancing protein extravasation. A recent study has tested directly this hypothesis. Eliceiri et al. [25] have shown that members of the Src family are differentially involved in mediating VEGF-dependent permeability versus angiogenesis. According to these studies, the vascular permeability-enhancing activity of VEGF specifically depends on Src or Yes [25]. Since mice lacking src and yes display a normal angiogenic response to VEGF, develop normally and do not show any overt defect in the vasculature, these finding imply that enhanced vascular permeability is not a requirement for VEGF-dependent angiogenesis.

VEGF Tyrosine Kinase Receptors

Two VEGF receptor tyrosine kinases are known, Flt-1 (VEGF-1) [26, 27] and KDR (VEGFR-2) [28]. Gene targeting studies have demonstrated that both Flt-1 and Flk-1/KDR are essential for development of the embryonic vasculature in mice [29, 30]. There is compelling evidence that Flt-1 and KDR have different signal transduction properties and possibly mediate different functions [31, 32]. Flk-1/KDR undergoes strong ligand-dependent tyrosine phosphorylation in intact cells and mediated mitogenesis and chemotaxis in response to VEGF, while Flt-1 reveals weak or undetectable responses [31, 32]. The generation of receptor-selective VEGF mutants has shown that only the mutants that bind KDR have mitogenic activity [33]. It has been suggested that Flt-1 is not primarily a signaling receptor but rather a 'decoy' receptor, able to regulate in a negative fashion the activity of VEGF on the vascular endothelium by sequestering and rendering this ligand less available to Flk-1/KDR [34]. Recent studies have provided evidence in support of such hypothesis. Hiratsuka et al. [35] have shown that a targeted mutation resulting in a Flt-1 receptor lacking the tyrosine kinase (TK) domain but able to bind VEGF does not result in lethality or any defect in embryonic development and angiogenesis in mice, while, as mentioned above, complete inactivation of the receptor results in early embryonic lethality. Endothelial cells isolated from Flt-1($TK^{-/-}$) animals display a normal mitogenic response to VEGF. Furthermore, a reexamination of the original Flt-1 knockout has revealed that the primary defect in Flt-$1^{-/-}$ embryos is an increase in the number of endothelial progenitors, leading to the previously described vascular disorganization [36]. Interestingly, a recent study has shown that the juxtamembrane region of Flt-1 constitutively inhibits VEGF-dependent endothelial cell migration and PI 3′ kinase activation [37]. Further mutational analysis shows that a short divergent sequence is responsible for such repressor function. However, mutant Flt-1 receptors that lack this sequence do not transmit effective proliferative signals, suggesting that this receptor function is regulated separately and that additional repressor elements exist. However, in some cell types other than endothelial cells, Flt-1 demonstrates evidence of biological activity, including the ability to mediate monocyte chemotaxis [38] and induce metalloproteinase expression in smooth muscle cells [39].

Neuropilin-1 as a Coreceptor for KDR

Soker et al. [40] have identified a receptor that binds VEGF165 but not VEGF121. This isoform-specific VEGF receptor is identical to human neuropilin-1 (NRP1) [41], a receptor for the collapsin/semaphorin family that mediates neuronal cell guidance by providing a repulsive cue to sensory growth cones [42]. When coexpressed in cells with KDR, NRP1enhanced the binding of VEGF165 to KDR and VEGF165-mediated chemotaxis. Conversely, inhibition of VEGF165 binding to NRP1 inhibits its binding to KDR and its mitogenic activity for endothelial cells. These findings suggest that neuropilin-1 may present VEGF165 to the KDR receptor in a manner that enhances the effectiveness of KDR-mediated signal transduction. Recently, Miao et al. [43] have shown that collapsin-1 binding to NRP1 can antagonize the chemotactic action of VEGF. These findings indicate that endothelial cells may respond to both positive and negative directional cues and reinforce the analogy between axon guidance processes and angiogenesis. Studies on the ephrins, a family of Eph receptor ligands previously implicated in neuronal patterning and neural cell guidance formation and more recently shown to be required for the development of the vascular system [44, 45], have also emphasized such molecular analogies.

Role of VEGF in Embryonic and Early Postnatal Angiogenesis

In 1996, two independent studies generated direct evidence for the role played by VEGF in embryonic vasculogenesis [46, 47]. Inactivation of a single VEGF allele in mice resulted in defective angiogenesis and embryonic lethality between day 11 and 12. Also, an isoform-specific knockout of the VEGF gene has been reported [48]. 50% of the mice that express exclusively VEGF120 died shortly after delivery, while the remainder died within 2 weeks. The survivors demonstrated impaired myocardial contractility, heart enlargement and defective angiogenesis leading to ischemic cardiomyopathy.

To selectively investigate the role of VEGF in the heart, Giordano et al. [49] performed a heart-specific VEGF knockout. Using Cre-*loxP* technology, mice with cardiomyocyte-specific deletion of the gene encoding VEGF were generated. Cardiac myocytes represent less than one third of the total cell number in the heart, yet knockout mice had reduced body weights and their hearts were thin walled, dilated, hypovascular and display definitive basal contractile dysfunction. These findings establish a critical role for the cardiac myocyte as a secretory cell.

Inducible, Cre-*loxP*-mediated gene targeting or administration of a soluble VEGF receptor chimeric protein [mFlt(1–3)-IgG] were used to inactivate VEGF in early postnatal life [50]. Mice containing the 'floxed' VEGF allele were bred to a strain transgenic for Cre recombinase controlled by an interferon-inducible promoter (MX-1) [51]. Partial inhibition of VEGF achieved by this inducible gene targeting system resulted in increased mortality, stunted body growth and impaired organ development, most notably of the liver. Administration of mFlt(1–3)-IgG, which achieves a considerably higher degree of VEGF inhibition, resulted in nearly complete growth arrest when the treatment was initiated at day 1 or day 8 postnatally. Such treatment was also accompanied by rapid lethality. Interestingly, the liver of mFlt(1–3)-IgG-treated neonates had fewer endothelial cells and focal loss of integrity of the space of Disse. Endothelial cells isolated from the liver of mFlt(1–3)-IgG-treated neonates demonstrated increased apoptotic index, indicating that VEGF is required not only for proliferation but also for survival of endothelial cells. However, VEGF inhibition resulted in less significant alterations as the animal matured and the dependence on VEGF was eventually lost sometime after the 4th postnatal week, indicating that a process of maturation occurs in endothelial cells such that they eventually lose their dependence on VEGF for survival.

Role of VEGF in Endochondral Bone Formation

Endochondral bone formation is a fundamental mechanism for longitudinal bone growth during vertebrate development [52]. Recently, the role of VEGF in endochondral bone formation has been examined. It has been shown that the VEGF mRNA is expressed by hypertrophic chondrocytes in the epiphyseal growth plate [53, 54]. Inhibition of VEGF activity using mFlt(1–3)-IgG resulted in nearly complete suppression of blood vessel invasion, concomitant with impaired trabecular bone formation. Although proliferation, differentiation and maturation of chondrocytes were apparently normal, resorption of hypertrophic chondrocytes was inhibited, resulting in a 3- to 6-fold expansion of the hypertrophic chondrocyte zone [53]. These findings indicate that VEGF-dependent blood vessels are essential for coupling cartilage resorption with bone formation. Therefore, the vasculature carries the essential cellular and humoral signals required for correct growth plate morphogenesis.

Role of VEGF in the Pathophysiology of the Female Reproductive Tract

Follicular growth and the development and endocrine function of the ovarian corpus luteum (CL) are dependent on the proliferation of new capillary vessels [55]. Subsequently, the blood vessels regress, suggesting the coordinated action of inducers and inhibitors of angiogenesis in the course of the ovarian cycle [56, 57]. Previous studies have shown the VEGF mRNA is temporally and spatially related to the proliferation of blood vessels in the rat, mouse and primate ovary and in the rat uterus [58–61]. The availability of an effective inhibitor of rodent VEGF, such as a truncated soluble Flt-1 receptor [mFlt(1–3)-IgG], has made it possible to determine the role of VEGF in such processes [62, 63]. Treatment with mFlt(1–3)-IgG resulted in virtually complete suppression of CL angiogenesis in a rat model of hormonally induced ovulation [63]. This effect was associated with inhibition of CL development and progesterone release. A similar inhibition of CL and uterine angiogenesis has been observed in cynomolgous monkeys treated with a humanized anti-VEGF monoclonal antibody (rhuMab VEGF) [64]. Furthermore, Fraser et al. [65] have recently shown that administration of an anti-VEGF neutralizing antibody also inhibits CL development in the marmoset. These findings support the notion that VEGF-mediated angiogenesis is essential for luteal function across species.

Several studies have examined the possible role of VEGF in the pathogenesis of ovarian hyperstimulation syndrome (OHSS). This potentially fatal condition may follow medical induction of ovulation with gonadotropins. Although the mechanisms that lead to the development of the syndrome are not clearly understood, two major aspects are ovarian enlargement, with multiple follicular cysts and corpora lutea, and increased vascular permeability, leading to extravasation of protein-rich fluid out of the intravascular space [66, 67]. According to McClure et al. [68] VEGF is the major capillary permeability agent in OHSS ascites fluid. Similarly, Levin et al. [69] have shown that follicular fluid from OHSS patients contains permeability-enhancing activity that can be blocked by anti-VEGF neutralizing antibodies. However, other studies have cast doubt on the hypothesis that VEGF may be a causative factor in the vascular permeability associated with OHSS. Kobayashi et al. [70] proposed the kallikrein-kinin system, rather than VEGF, is primarily responsible for such increased permeability. It is possible that, while VEGF alone is insufficient to cause the symptoms of OHSS, it may synergize with a number of inflammatory cytokines, including IL-2 and IL-6, that are known to be elevated as well [71] and thus blocking VEGF may have a therapeutic value in this condition.

Role of VEGF in Tumor Angiogenesis

The observation that tumor growth is accompanied by blood vessel proliferation was made over a century ago. In 1939, Ide et al. [72] employing a transparent chamber implanted in the rabbit ear, which enables a direct in vivo visualization, demonstrated that the growth of tumor xenografts is accompanied by new vessel growth, making the authors hypothesize that such neovascularization facilitates tumor growth by delivering nutrients and oxygen and removing catabolic products. These hypotheses were considerably furthered in 1945 by Algire and Chalkley [73] who applied for the first time a quantitative approach to assess tumor-associated neovascularization. The observation that the phase of rapid tumor growth is preceded by a local increase in blood vessel density led these authors to conclude that 'the rapid growth of tumor explants is dependent upon the development of a rich vascular supply' [73]. In the early 1970s, Folkman [74] proposes that antiangiogenesis could be an effective strategy to treat cancer and initiated experimental work aimed toward the purification of tumor angiogenic factors. Clearly, a major problem in the field was the identification of the mediators of tumor-associated angiogenesis.

In 1993 Kim et al. [5] reported that anti-VEGF monoclonal antibodies substantially inhibit the growth of human tumor xenografts in immunodeficient mice. These findings provided the first direct evidence in support of the hypothesis that tumor growth is angiogenesis-dependent. There is now compelling evidence that VEGF is indeed a major tumor angiogenesis factor. The VEGF mRNA is upregulated in a large number of human tumor types [for reviews, see 1, 22]. There is also a substantial body of data documenting that inhibition of VEGF activity results in the suppression of growth of a wide variety of tumor cell lines in murine models [8]. A recent study has shown that combining an anti-Flk-1/KDR antibody with low-dose vinblastin results in a greater inhibitory activity in murine models of neuroblastoma than either treatment alone [75].

Clinical trials in cancer patients are ongoing with several VEGF inhibitors, including a rhuMab VEGF [76], an anti-KDR antibody [77] and various small molecules inhibiting KDR signal transduction [78–80].

Phase II clinical data, presented in May 2000 at the Annual Meeting of the American Society of Clinical Oncology, provided initial evidence that rhuMab VEGF, in combination with conventional chemotherapy, results in an increase in time to progression in patients with non-small-cell lung [81] as well as metastatic colorectal [82] carcinoma and may also increase survival. Furthermore, rhuMab VEGF administered as a single agent to patients with relapsed metastatic breast cancer shows evidence of clinical efficacy [83]. Also, a phase I/II with SU5416, a small molecule inhibitor of KDR has shown preliminary evidence of activity in patients with metastatic colorectal cancer [84]. Phase III studies are currently underway to confirm and fully assess the benefit of these anti-VEGF treatments in patients with advanced cancer.

Role of VEGF in Hematopoiesis and Hematological Malignancies

As previously indicated, knockout experiments targeting VEGF [46, 47] and KDR/Flk-1 [30] revealed severe decreases in the numbers of angioblasts, the precursor for endothelial cells as well as in the amounts of total hematopoietic progenitors derived from mesenchymal progenitors. Recently, VEGF was found to be produced by hematopoietic stem cells (HSCs) in response to cytokine stimulation [85] and KDR was identified on a subset of multipotent human HSCs [30, 86]. Both, in long-term in vitro culture assays and in surrogate in vivo models, pluripotent stem cell activity segregated with KDR expression. CD34+, KDR+ progenitor cells displayed pluripotent activity, whereas the CD34+, KDR– fraction contained only committed progenitors [87]. In adult mice, the effects of prolonged systemic administration of VEGF on hematopoiesis was characterized by intense medullary hyperplasia of immature myeloid elements and arrest of erythroid maturation [88]. These experiments established that VEGF and KDR are essential for hematopoiesis. However, the molecular mechanism underlying the HSC differentiation and survival remained elusive.

Hematological malignancies often result from an impaired control of early HSC survival [89]. Leukemias originate from HSC at different stages of their maturation and differentiation. Acute leukemias originate from immature HSCs that have the capacity to undergo self-renewal, whereas chronic leukemias seem to originate from the more mature, committed hematopoietic progenitor cells. VEGF and both its receptors were found to be upregulated in many human hematopoietic tumor cell lines and tumor tissues representing multiple lineages and diseases, including leukemia, lymphoma and multiple myeloma [90–92]. In these studies, it was found that VEGF is overexpressed in 72% of acute myelogenous leukemia specimens and the corresponding expression of Flt-1 and KDR message in 52 and 19% of patients, respectively [92]. Similar frequencies were found in studies conducted by Bellamy et al. [91] where an overall 82% of acute myelogenous leukemia patients displayed increased VEGF levels, and 76% had Flt-1 upregulated but no increase in KDR positivity was found. In patients suffering from the less aggressive myelodysplastic syndrome, 76% had elevated VEGF levels, 69% had increase Flt-1 and 19% increased KDR expression. Interestingly, upregulation of VEGF in myelodysplastic syndrome might reflect the high frequency of mutant *ras* activation, which is recognized to induce transcriptional activation of VEGF gene expression [93]. Di Raimondo et al. [94] have recently measured the levels of VEGF, as well as bFGF and HFG, in multiple myeloma patients and found that the concentrations of these factors parallels the activity of disease. Interestingly, higher levels of these angiogenic factors were in the bone marrow compared to peripheral blood, suggesting that bone marrow microenvironment is their major source. In summary, these finding suggested that the production of VEGF by malignant myeloid precursors might serve both, as an autocrine growth stimulus and a diffusible paracrine signal mediating the local generation of growth factors that foster leukemia survival and self-renewal.

Recent studies have shown that leukemic cells are capable of producing other members of the VEGF gene family such as VEGF-C and possibly VEGF-D [92]. These molecules are thought to signal also through KDR. In conclusion, inhibition of VEGF or VEGF receptor activity in nonsolid tumors such as leukemias might represent a highly effective strategy to inhibit tumor growth and metastasis, since it potentially interferes with two hallmarks of tumor progression, angiogenesis and leukemia cell proliferation.

Role of VEGF in Other Pathological Conditions

Neovascularization is a major cause of visual loss also in proliferative diabetic retinopathy and age-related macular degeneration (AMD), the overall leading cause of blindness [95]. The VEGF levels are elevated in the eye fluids of patients with ischemic retinal disease [6] and VEGF blockade results in suppression of ischemia-induced retinal neovascularization in animal models [7]. Several studies have also demonstrated the immunohistochemical localization of VEGF in surgically resected choroidal neovascular membranes from AMD patients [96, 97]. These findings suggest a role for VEGF in the progression of AMD-related choroidal neovascularization. Clinical trials using intraocular administration of a high affinity of humanized anti-VEGF Fab [98] are currently in phase I.

Recently, van Bruggen et al. [99] tested the hypothesis that VEGF inhibition achieved by administration of mFlt(1–3)-IgG may have beneficial effects in cortical ischemia. Using high-resolution magnetic resonance imaging techniques to quantify the extent of the edematous changes, a significant reduction in the volume of the edematous tissue was observed 1 day following the onset of ischemia in a murine model. Further, measurements of the resultant infarct size, measured several weeks later, revealed a significant sparing of cortical tissue in the mFlt(1–3)-IgG-treated group. These results demonstrate that antagonism of VEGF reduces ischemic-reperfusion-related brain edema and injury and raise the possibility that VEGF inhibition may play a role in the prevention of the sequelae of brain edema.

Perspectives

The role of VEGF in developmental and pathological angiogenesis is well established. Yet, numerous fundamental questions remain to be fully answered, such as the significance of the Flt-1 receptor. The recent finding that key signaling functions in Flt-1 are constitutively inhibited by repressor motifs emphasizes the unique characteristics of this receptor [37] An important issue is also the significance of other members of the VEGF family that bind selectively Flt-1 such as PlGF [34] and VEGF-B [100]. Recent studies indicate that VEGF-B inactivation in mice results in reduced heart size and impaired recovery from experimentally induced myocardial ischemia, although the animals develop normally and fail to display any overt deficit [101]. These findings suggest a significant albeit not essential role in the modulation of coronary angiogenesis.

The possibility that VEGF may be used to promote revascularization in myocardial or limb ischemia has received a great deal of attention [8]. So far, the clinical results have been inconclusive, due to the small sample size, or frankly disappointing. A placebo-controlled phase II trial in patients with coronary ischemia did not show evidence of clinical benefit following intracoronary and intravenous administration of recombinant VEGF [102]. Even bFGF, a potent angiogenic molecule that also raised considerable expectations, has failed to demonstrate any significant benefit in coronary ischemia patients in a large placebo-controlled trial [Simons, pers. commun.]. As previously discussed, several factors may account for the discrepancy between the remarkable efficacy of both molecules in various animal models and the clinical results [8]. Currently, several laboratories are exploring the possibility that a more persistent exposure to VEGF than that achieved in the earlier clinical trial [102] as well as the combination with other factors may achieve better results. Also, other potential clinical applications of VEGF-induced angiogenesis are receiving attention. For example, on the basis of the key role played by VEGF in bone angiogenesis and endochondral bone formation [53], it is conceivable that application of this factor may be useful to enhance revascularization in orthopedic conditions like nonhealing fractures. In this context, a recent study has shown that local VEGF administration may induce ossification of a fibrocartilaginous reunion created by rapid distraction [103], suggesting that VEGF may be used for the treatment of avascular nonunions.

Finally, over the next two or three years, several large clinical studies should provide a conclusive answer to the question of whether targeting the VEGF system is a valid approach to treat cancer and other disorders such as AMD.

References

1 Ferrara N, Davis-Smyth T: The biology of vascular endothelial growth factor. Endocr Rev 1997;18:4–25.
2 Ferrara N: Role of vascular endothelial growth factor in the regulation of angiogenesis. Kidney Int 1999;56:794–814.
3 Korpelainen EI, Alitalo K: Signaling angiogenesis and lymphangiogenesis. Curr Opin Cell Biol 1998;10:159–164.
4 Leung DW, Cachianes G, Kuang WJ, Goeddel DV, Ferrara N: Vascular endothelial growth factor is a secreted angiogenic mitogen. Science 1989;246:1306–1309.
5 Kim KJ, Li B, Winer J, Armanini M, Gillett N, Phillips HS, Ferrara N: Inhibition of vascular endothelial growth factor-induced angiogenesis suppresses tumor growth in vivo. Nature 1993; 362:841–844.
6 Aiello LP, Avery RL, Arrigg PG, Keyt BA, Jampel HD, Shah ST, Pasquale LR, Thieme H, Iwamoto MA, Park JE, Nguyen H, Aiello LM, Ferrara N, King GL: Vascular endothelial growth factor in ocular fluid of patients with diabetic retinopathy and other retinal disorders. N Engl J Med 1994;331:1480–1487.
7 Aiello LP, Pierce EA, Foley ED, Takagi H, Chen H, Riddle L, Ferrara N, King GL, Smith LE: Suppression of retinal neovascularization in vivo by inhibition of vascular endothelial growth factor (VEGF) using soluble VEGF-receptor chimeric proteins. Proc Natl Acad Sci USA 1995;92:10457–10461.
8 Ferrara N, Alitalo K: Clinical applications of angiogenic growth factors and their inhibitors. Nat Med 1999;5:1359–1364.
9 Ferrara N, Henzel WJ: Pituitary follicular cells secrete a novel heparin-binding growth factor specific for vascular endothelial cells. Biochem Biophys Res Commun 1989;161:851–858.
10 Conn G, Bayne ML, Soderman DD, Kwok PW, Sullivan KA, Palisi TM, Hope DA, Thomas KA: Amino acid and cDNA sequences of a vascular endothelial cell mitogen that is homologous to platelet-derived growth factor. Proc Natl Acad Sci USA 1990;87:2628–2632.
11 Plouet J, Schilling J, Gospodarowicz D: Isolation and characterization of a newly identified endothelial cell mitogen produced by AtT20 cells. EMBO J 1989;8:3801–3808.
12 Guerrin M, Moukadiri H, Chollet P, Moro F, Dutt K, Malecaze F, Plouet J: Vasculotropin/vascular endothelial growth factor is an autocrine growth factor for human retinal pigment epithelial cells cultured in vitro. J Cell Physiol 1995;164:385–394.
13 Oberg-Welsh C, Sandler S, Andersson A, Welsh M: Effects of vascular endothelial growth factor on pancreatic duct cell replication and the insulin production of fetal islet-like cell clusters in vitro. Mol Cell Endocrinol 1997;126:125–132.
14 Sondell M, Lundborg G, Kanje M: Vascular endothelial growth factor has neurotrophic activity and stimulates axonal outgrowth, enhancing cell survival and Schwann cell proliferation in the peripheral nervous system. J Neurosci 1999;19:5731–5740.
15 Alon T, Hemo I, Itin A, Pe'er J, Stone J, Keshet E: Vascular endothelial growth factor acts as a survival factor for newly formed retinal vessels and has implications for retinopathy of prematurity. Nat Med 1995;1:1024–1028.

16 Gerber HP, Dixit V, Ferrara N: Vascular endothelial growth factor induces expression of the antiapoptotic proteins Bcl-2 and A1 in vascular endothelial cells. J Biol Chem 1998;273: 13313–13316.
17 Gerber HP, McMurtrey A, Kowalski, J, Yan M, Keyt BA, Dixit V, Ferrara N: VEGF regulates endothelial cell survival by the PI 3′-kinase/Akt signal transduction pathway. Requirement for Flk-1/KDR activation. J Biol Chem 1998;273:30336–30343.
18 Benjamin LE, Golijanin D, Itin A, Pode, D, Keshet E: Selective ablation of immature blood vessels in established human tumors follows vascular endothelial growth factor withdrawal. J Clin Invest 1999;103:159–165.
19 Yuan F, Chen Y, Dellian M, Safabakhsh N, Ferrara N, Jain RK: Time-dependent vascular regression and permeability changes in established human tumor xenografts induced by an anti-vascular endothelial growth factor/vascular permeability factor antibody. Proc Natl Acad Sci USA 1996;93:14765–14770.
20 Carmeliet P, Lampugnani MG, Moons L, Breviario F, Compernolle V, Bono F, Balconi G, Spagnuolo R, Oostuyse B, Dewerchin M, Zanetti A, Angellilo A, Mattot V, Nuyens D, Lutgens E, Clotman F, de Ruiter MC, Gittenberger-de Groot A, Poelmann R, Lupu F, Herbert JM, Collen D, Dejana E: Targeted deficiency or cytosolic truncation of the VE-cadherin gene in mice impairs VEGF-mediated endothelial survival and angiogenesis. Cell 1999;98:147–157.
21 Senger DR, Galli SJ, Dvorak AM, Perruzzi CA, Harvey VS, Dvorak HF: Tumor cells secrete a vascular permeability factor that promotes accumulation of ascites fluid. Science 1983;219: 983–985.
22 Dvorak HF, Brown LF, Detmar M, Dvorak AM: Vascular permeability factor/vascular endothelial growth factor, microvascular hyperpermeability, and angiogenesis. Am J Pathol 1995;146:1029–1039.
23 Dvorak HF: Tumors: Wounds that do not heal. Similarities between tumor stroma generation and wound healing. N Engl J Med 1986;315: 1650–1659.
24 Dvorak HF, Harvey VS, Estrella P, Brown LF, McDonagh J, Dvorak AM: Fibrin containing gels induce angiogenesis: Implications for tumor stroma generation and wound healing. Lab Invest 1987;57:673–686.
25 Eliceiri BP, Paul R, Schwartzberg PL, Hood JD, Leng J, Cheresh DA: Selective requirement for Src kinases during VEGF-induced angiogenesis and vascular permeability. Mol Cell 1999;4:915–924.
26 Shibuya M, Yamaguchi S, Yamane A, Ikeda T, Tojo A, Matsushime H, Sato M: Nucleotide sequence and expression of a novel human receptor-type tyrosine kinase (flt) closely related to the fms family. Oncogene 1990;8:519–527.
27 de Vries C, Escobedo JA, Ueno H, Houck K, Ferrara N, Williams LT: The fms-like tyrosine kinase, a receptor for vascular endothelial growth factor. Science 1992;255:989–991.
28 Terman BI, Dougher Vermazen M, Carrion ME, Dimitrov D, Armellino DC, Gospodarowicz D, Bohlen P: Identification of the KDR tyrosine kinase as a receptor for vascular endothelial cell growth factor. Biochem Biophys Res Commun 1992;187:1579–1586.
29 Fong GH, Rossant J, Gertsenstein M, Breitman ML: Role of the Flt-1 receptor tyrosine kinase in regulating the assembly of vascular endothelium. Nature 1995;376:66–70.
30 Shalaby F, Rossant J, Yamaguchi TP, Gertsenstein M, Wu XF, Breitman ML, Schuh AC: Failure of blood-island formation and vasculogenesis in Flk-1-deficient mice. Nature 1995; 376:62–66.
31 Waltenberger J, Claesson Welsh L, Siegbahn A, Shibuya M, Heldin CH: Different signal transduction properties of KDR and Flt1, two receptors for vascular endothelial growth factor. J Biol Chem 1994;269:26988–26995.
32 Seetharam L, Gotoh N, Maru Y, Neufeld G, Yamaguchi S, Shibuya M: A unique signal transduction from FLT tyrosine kinase, a receptor for vascular endothelial growth factor VEGF. Oncogene 1995;10:135–147.
33 Keyt BA, Nguyen HV, Berleau LT, Duarte CM, Park J, Chen H, Ferrara N: Identification of vascular endothelial growth factor determinants for binding KDR and FLT-1 receptors. Generation of receptor-selective VEGF variants by site-directed mutagenesis. J Biol Chem 1996;271:5638–5646.
34 Park JE, Chen HH, Winer J, Houck KA, Ferrara N: Placenta growth factor. Potentiation of vascular endothelial growth factor bioactivity, in vitro and in vivo, high affinity binding to Flt-1 but not to Flk-1/KDR. J Biol Chem 1994; 269:25646–25654.
35 Hiratsuka S, Minowa O, Kuno J, Noda T, Shibuya M: Flt-1 lacking the tyrosine kinase domain is sufficient for normal development and angiogenesis in mice. Proc Natl Acad Sci USA 1998;4:9349–9354.
36 Fong GH, Zhang L, Bryce DM, Peng J: Increased hemangioblast commitment, not vascular disorganization, is the primary defect in flt-1 knock-out mice. Development 1999;126: 3015–3025.
37 Gille H, Kowalski J, Yu L, Chen H, Pisabarro MT, Davis-Smyth T, Ferrara N: A repressor sequence in the juxtamembrane domain of Flt-1 (VEGFR-1) constitutively inhibits VEGF-dependent PI 3 kinase activation and endothelial cell migration. EMBO J 2000;19:4064–4073.
38 Barleon B, Sozzani S, Zhou D, Weich HA, Mantovani A, Marme D: Migration of human monocytes in response to vascular endothelial growth factor (VEGF) is mediated via the VEGF receptor flt-1. Blood 1996;87:3336–3343.
39 Wang H, Keiser JA: Vascular endothelial growth factor upregulates the expression of matrix metalloproteinases in vascular smooth muscle cells: Role of flt-1. Circ Res 1998;83: 832–840.
40 Soker S, Takashima S, Miao HQ, Neufeld G, Klagsbrun M: Neuropilin-1 is expressed by endothelial and tumor cells as an isoform-specific receptor for vascular endothelial growth factor. Cell 1998;92:735–745.
41 Fujisawa H, Kitsukawa T: Receptors for collapsin/semaphorins. Curr Opin Neurobiol 1998;8:587–592.
42 Luo Y, Jan LY, Jan YN: Collapsin: A protein in brain that induces collapse and paralysis of neuronal growth cones. Cell 1993;75:217–227.
43 Miao HQ, Soker S, Feiner L, Alonso JL, Raper JA, Klagsbrun M: Neuropilin-1 mediates collapsin-1/semaphorin III inhibition of endothelial cell motility: Functional competition of collapsin-1 and vascular endothelial growth factor-165. J Cell Biol 1999;146:233–242.
44 Wang HU, Chen ZF, Anderson DJ: Molecular distinction and angiogenic interaction between embryonic arteries and veins revealed by ephrin-B2 and its receptor Eph-B4. Cell 1998;93: 741–753.
45 Adams RH, Wilkinson GA, Weiss C, Diella F, Gale NW, Deutsch U, Risau W, Klein R: Roles of ephrinB ligands and EphB receptors in cardiovascular development: Demarcation of arterial/venous domains, vascular morphogenesis, sprouting angiogenesis. Genes Dev 1999; 13:295–306.
46 Carmeliet P, Ferreira V, Breier G, Pollefeyt S, Kieckens L, Gertsenstein M, Fahrig M, Vandenhoeck A, Harpal K, Eberhardt C, Declercq C, Pawling J, Moons L, Collen D, Risau W, Nagy A: Abnormal blood vessel development and lethality in embryos lacking a single VEGF allele. Nature 1996;380:435–439.
47 Ferrara N, Carver Moore K, Chen H, Dowd M, Lu L, O'Shea KS, Powell Braxton L, Hillan KJ, Moore MW: Heterozygous embryonic lethality induced by targeted inactivation of the VEGF gene. Nature 1996;380:439–442.
48 Carmeliet P, Ng Y-S, Nuyens D, Theilmeier G, Brusselmans K, Cornelissen I, Ehler E, Kakkar VV, Stalmans I, Mattot V, Perriard J-C, Dewerchin M, Flameng W, Nagy A, Lupu F, Moons L, Collen D, D'Amore PA, Shima DT: Impaired myocardial angiogenesis and ischemic cardiomyopathy in mice lacking the vascular endothelila growth factor isoforms VEGF164 and VEGF188. Nat Med 1999;5: 495–502.
49 Giordano FJ, Gerber HP, Williams SP, VanBruggen N, Bunting S, Ruiz-Lozano PY, Gu Y, Hickey R, Nath AK, Dalton N, Peterson KL, Ross J, Chien KR, Ferrara N: A cardiac myocyte VEGF paracrine pathway is required to maintain cardiac function. Proc Natl Acad Sci USA 2001;98:5780–5785.
50 Gerber HP, Hillan KJ, Ryan AM, Kowalski J, Keller G-A, Rangell L, Wright BD, Radtke F, Aguet M, Ferrara N: VEGF is required for growth and survival in neonatal mice. Development 1999;126:1149–1159.
51 Kuhn R, Schwenk F, Aguet M, Rajewsky K: Inducible gene targeting in mice. Science 1995; 269:1427–1429.
52 Poole AR: Cartilage: Molecular Aspects. Boca Raton, CRC Press, 1991, pp 179–211.

53 Gerber HP, Vu TH, Ryan AM, Kowalski J, Werb Z, Ferrara N: VEGF couples hypertrophic cartilage remodeling, ossification and angiogenesis during endochondral bone formation. Nat Med 1999;5:623–628.
54 Carlevaro MF, Cermelli S, Cancedda R, Descalzi Cancedda F: Vascular endothelial growth factor (VEGF) in cartilage neovascularization and chondrocyte differentiation: Auto-paracrine role during endochondral bone formation. J Cell Sci 2000;113:59–69.
55 Bassett DL: The changes in the vascular pattern of the ovary of the albino rat during the estrous cycle. Am J Anat 1943;73:251–278.
56 Goede V, Schmidt T, Kimmina S, Kozian D, Augustin HG: Analysis of blood vessel maturation processes during cyclic ovarian angiogenesis. Lab Invest 1998;78:1385–1394.
57 Maisonpierre PC, Suri C, Jones PF, Bartunkova S, Wiegend SJ, Radziejewski C, Compton D, McClain J, Aldrich TH, Papadopulos N, Daly TJ, Davis S, Sato TN, Yancopoulos GD: Angiopoietin-2, a natural antagonist for Tie-2 that disrupts in vivo angiogenesis. Science 1997;277:55–60.
58 Phillips HS, Hains J, Leung DW, Ferrara N: Vascular endothelial growth factor is expressed in rat corpus luteum. Endocrinology 1990;127: 965–967.
59 Ravindranath N, Little-Ihrig L, Phillips HS, Ferrara N, Zeleznik AJ: Vascular endothelial growth factor messenger ribonucleic acid expression in the primate ovary. Endocrinology 1992;131:254–260.
60 Shweiki D, Itin A, Neufeld G, Gitay-Goren H, Keshet E: Patterns of expression of vascular endothelial growth factor (VEGF) and VEGF receptors in mice suggest a role in hormonally-mediated angiogenesis. J Clin Invest 1993;91: 2235–2243.
61 Cullinan-Bove K, Koos RD: Vascular endothelial growth factor/vascular permeability factor expression in the rat uterus: Rapid stimulation by estrogen correlates with estrogen-induced increases in uterine capillary permeability and growth. Endocrinology 1993;133:829–837.
62 Davis-Smyth T, Chen H, Park J, Presta LG, Ferrara N: The second immunoglobulin-like domain of the VEGF tyrosine kinase receptor Flt-1 determines ligand binding and may initiate a signal transduction cascade. EMBO J 1996;15:4919–4927.
63 Ferrara N, Chen H, Davis-Smyth T, Gerber H-P, Nguyen T-N, Peers D, Chisholm V, Hillan KJ, Schwall RH: Vascular endothelial growth factor is essential for corpus luteum angiogenesis. Nat Med 1998;4:336–340.
64 Ryan AM, Eppler DB, Hagler KE, Bruner RH, Thomford PJ, Hall RL, Shopp GM, O'Neill CA: Preclinical safety evaluation of rhuMAb VEGF, an antiangiogenic humanized monoclonal antibody. Toxicol Pathol 1999;27:78–86.
65 Fraser HM, Dickson SE, Lunn SF, Wulff C, Morris KD, Carroll VA, Bicknell R: Suppression of luteal angiogenesis in the primate after neutralization of vascular endothelial growth factor. Endocrinology 2000;141:995–1000.
66 Engel T, Jewelewicz R, Dyrenfurth I, Speroff L, Vande Wiele RL: Ovarian hyperstimulation syndrome: Report of one case with notes on pathogenesis and treatment. Am J Obstet Gynecol 1972;112:1052–1057.
67 Haning RJ, Strawn E, Nolten W: Pathophysiology of the ovarian hyperstimulation syndrome. Obstet Gynecol 1985;166:220–224.
68 McClure N, Healy DL, Rogers PA, Sullivan J, Beaton L, Haning RV, Connolly DT, Robertson DM: Vascular endothelial growth factor as a capillary permeability agent in ovarian hyperstimulation syndrome. Lancet 1994;344:235–269.
69 Levin ER, Rosen GF, Cassidenti DL, Yee B, Meldrum D, Wisot A, Pedram A: Role of vascular endothelial cell growth factor in ovarian hyperstimulation syndrome. J Clin Invest 1998;102:1978–1985.
70 Kobayashi H, Okada Y, Asahina T, Gotoh J, Terao T: The kallikrein-kinin system, but not vascular endothelial growth factor, plays a role in the increased vascular permeability associated with ovarian hyperstimulation syndrome. J Mol Endocrinol 1998;20:363–374.
71 Aboulghar MA, Mansour RT, Serour GI, El Helw BA, Shaarawy M: Elevated levels of interleukin-2, soluble interleukin-2 receptor alpha, interleukin-6, soluble interleukin-6 receptor and vascular endothelial growth factor in serum and ascitic fluid of patients with severe ovarian hyperstimulation syndrome. Eur J Obstet Gynecol 1999;87:81–85.
72 Ide AG, Baker NH, Warren SL: Vascularization of the Brown Pearce rabbit epithelioma transplant as seen in the transparent ear chamber. Am J Roentgenol 1939;42:891–899.
73 Algire GH, Chalkley HW: Vascular reactions of normal and malignant tissues in vivo. I. Vascular reactions of mice to wounds and to normal and neoplastic transplants. J Natl Cancer Inst 1945;6:73–85.
74 Folkman J: Tumor angiogenesis: Therapeutic implications. N Engl J Med 1971;285:1182–1186.
75 Klement G, Baruchel S, Rak J, Man S, Clark K, Hicklin DJ, Bohlen P, Kerbel RS: Continuous low-dose therapy with vinblastine and VEGF receptor-2 antibody induces sustained tumor regression without overt toxicity. J Clin Invest 2000;105:R15–24.
76 Presta LG, Chen H, O'Connor SJ, Chisholm V, Meng YG, Krummen L, Winkler M, Ferrara N: Humanization of an anti-VEGF monoclonal antibody for the therapy of solid tumors and other disorders. Cancer Res 1997;57:4593–4599.
77 Prewett M, Huber J, Li Y, Santiago A, O'Connor W, King K, Overholser J, Hooper A, Pytowski B, Witte L, Bohlen P, Hicklin DJ: Antivascular endothelial growth factor receptor (fetal liver kinase 1) monoclonal antibody inhibits tumor angiogenesis. Cancer Res 1999;59: 5209–5218.
78 Strawn LM, McMahon G, App H, Schreck R, Kuchler WR, Longhi MP, Hui TH, Tang C, Levitzki A, Gazit A, Chen I, Keri G, Orfi L, Risau W, Flamme I, Ullrich A, Hirth KP, Shawver LK: Flk-1 as a target for tumor growth inhibition. Cancer Res 1996;56:3540–3545.
79 Wood JM, Bold G, Buchdunger E, Cozens R, Ferrari S, Frei J, Hofmann F, Mestan J, Mett H, O'Reilly T, Persohn E, Rosel J, Schnell C, Stover D, Theuer A, Towbin H, Wenger F, Woods-Cook K, Menrad A, Siemeister G, Schirner M, Thierauch KH, Schneider MR, Drevs J, Martiny-Baron G, Totzke F: PTK787/ZK 222584, a novel and potent inhibitor of vascular endothelial growth factor receptor tyrosine kinases, impairs vascular endothelial growth factor-induced responses and tumor growth after oral administration. Cancer Res 2000;60:2178–2189.
80 Wedge SR, Ogilvie DJ, Dukes M, Kendrew J, Curwen JO, Hennequin LF, Thomas AP, Stokes ES, Curry B, Richmond GH, Wadsworth PF: ZD4190: An orally active inhibitor of vascular endothelial growth factor signaling with broad-spectrum antitumor efficacy. Cancer Res 2000;60:970–975.
81 DeVore R, Herbst RS, Langer CJ, Kelly K, Gaudreault J, Holmgren E, Novotny WF, Kabbinavar FA: A randomized Phase II Trial Comparing rhuMAb VEGF (Recombinant Humanized Monoclonal Antibody to Vascular Endothelial Cell Growth Factor) plus Carboplatin/Paclitaxel (CP) to CP Alone in Patients with Stage IIIB/IV NSCLC. 36th Annual Meeting of the American Society of Clinical Oncology, New Orleans, 2000.
82 Bergsland E, Fehrenbacher L, Meropol NJ, Novotny WF, Gaudreault J, Lieberman GFK: A Randomized Phase II Trial Comparing rhuMAb VEGF (Recombinant Humanized Monoclonal Antibody to Vascular Endothelial Cell Growth Factor) plus 5-Fluorouracil/Leucovorin (FU/LV) to FU/LV Alone in Patients with Metastatic Colorectal Cancer. 36th Annual Meeting of the American Society of Clinical Oncology, New Orleans, 2000.
83 Sledge G, Miller K, Novotny W, Gaudreault J, Ash M, Colbeigh M: A Phase II Trial of Single-Agent rhuMAb VEGF (Recombinant Humanized Monoclonal Antibody to Vascular Endothelila Growth Factor) in Patients with Relapsing Metastatic Breast Cancer. 36th Annual Meeting of the American Society of Clinical Oncology, New Orleans, 2000.
84 Rosen PJ, Amado R, Hecht JR, Chang D, Mulay M, Parson M, Laxa B, Brown J, Cropp G, Hannah A, Rosen L: A Phase I/II Study of SU5416 in Combination with 5-FU/Leucovorin in Patients with Metastatic Colorectal Cancer. 36th Annual Meeting of the American Society of Clinical Oncology, New Orleans, 2000.
85 Bautz F, Rafii S, Kanz L, Mohle R: Expression and secretion of vascular endothelial growth factor-A by cytokine-stimulated hematopoietic progenitor cells. Possible role in the hematopoietic microenvironment. Exp Hematol 2000; 28:700–706.

86 Kabrun N, Buhring HJ, Choi K, Ullrich A, Risau W, Keller G: Flk-1 expression defines a population of early embryonic hematopoietic precursors. Development 1997;124:2039–2048.
87 Ziegler BL, Valtieri M, Porada GA, De Maria R, Muller R, Masella B, Gabbianelli M, Casella I, Pelosi E, Bock T, Zanjani ED, Peschle C: KDR receptor: A key marker defining hematopoietic stem cells. Science 1999;285:1553–1558.
88 Gabrilovich D, Ishida T, Oyama T, Ran S, Kravtsov V, Nadaf S, Carbone DP: Vascular endothelial growth factor inhibits the development of dendritic cells and dramatically affects the differentiation of multiple hematopoietic lineages in vivo. Blood 1998;92:4150–4166.
89 Dias S, Hattori K, Zhu Z, Heissig B, Choy M, Lane W, Wu Y, Chadburn A, Hyjek E, Gill M, Hicklin DJ, Witte L, Moore MA, Rafii S: Autocrine stimulation of VEGFR-2 activates human leukemic cell growth and migration. J Clin Invest 2000;106:511–521.
90 Bellamy WT, Richter L, Frutiger Y, Grogan TM: Expression of vascular endothelial growth factor and its receptors in hematopoietic malignancies. Cancer Res 1999;59:728–733.
91 Bellamy WT, Richter L, Sirjani D, Roxas C, Glinsmann-Gibson B, Frutiger Y, Grogan TM, List AF: Vascular endothelial cell growth factor is an autocrine promoter of abnormal localized immature myeloid precursors and leukemia progenitor formation in myelodysplastic syndromes. Blood 2001;97:1427–1434.
92 Fielder W, Graeven U, Ergun S, Verago S, Kilic N, Stockschlader M, Hossfeld DK: Expression of FLT4 and its ligand VEGF-C in acute myeloid leukemia. Leukemia 1997;11:1234–1237.
93 Grugel S, Finkenzeller G, Weindel K, Barleon B, Marme D: Both v-Ha-Ras and v-Raf stimulate expression of the vascular endothelial growth factor in NIH 3T3 cells. J Biol Chem 1995;270:25915–25919.
94 Di Raimondo F, Azzaro MP, Palumbo GA, Bagnato S, Giustolisi G, Floridia P, Sortino G, Giustolisi R: Angiogenic factors in multiple myeloma: Higher levels in bone marrow than in peripheral blood. Haematologica 2000;85: 800–805.
95 Garner A: Vascular Diseases, ed 2. New York, Dekker, 1994.
96 Lopez PF, Sippy BD, Lambert HM, Thach AB, Hinton DR: Transdifferentiated retinal pigment epithelial cells are immunoreactive for vascular endothelial growth factor in surgically excised age-related macular degeneration-related choroidal neovascular membranes. Invest Ophthalmol Vis Sci 1996;37:855–868.
97 Kvanta A, Algvere PV, Berglin L, Seregard S: Subfoveal fibrovascular membranes in age-related macular degeneration express vascular endothelial growth factor. Invest Ophthalmol Vis Sci 1996;37:1929–1934.
98 Chen Y, Wiesmann C, Fuh G, Li B, Christinger HW, McKay P, de Vos AM, Lowman HB: Selection and analysis of an optimized anti-VEGF antibody: Crystal structure of an affinity-matured Fab in complex with antigen. J Mol Biol 1999;293:865–881.
99 van Bruggen N, Thibodeaux H, Palmer JT, Cairns B, Tumas D, Gerlai R, Williams S-P, van Lookeren Campagne M, Ferrara N: VEGF antagonism reduces cerebral edema formation and tissue damage following ischemic-reperfusion injury in the mouse brain. J Clin Invest 1999;104:1613–1620.
100 Olofsson B, Korpelainen E, Pepper MS, Mandriota SJ, Aase K, Kumar V, Gunji Y, Jeltsch MM, Shibuya M, Alitalo K, Eriksson U: Vascular endothelial growth factor B (VEGF-B) binds to VEGF receptor-1 and regulates plasminogen activator activity in endothelial cells. Proc Natl Acad Sci USA 1998;95: 11709–11714.
101 Bellomo D, Headrick JP, Silins GU, Paterson CA, Thomas PS, Gartside M, Mould A, Cahill MM, Tonks ID, Grimmond SM, Townson S, Wells C, Little M, Cummings MC, Hayward NK, Kay GF: Mice lacking the vascular endothelial growth factor-B gene (Vegfb) have smaller hearts, dysfunctional coronary vasculature, impaired recovery from cardiac ischemia. Circ Res 2000;86: E29–35.
102 Henry T, Annex BH, Azrin MA, McKendall GR, Willerson JT, Hendel RC, Giordano FJ, Klein R, Gibson CM, Berman DS, Luce CA, McCluskey ER: Double Blind, Placebo Controlled Trial of Recombinant Human Vascular Endothelial Growth Factor: The VIVA Trial. J Am Coll Cardiol 1999;33/2(suppl A):384A, 874.
103 Ogilvie C, Lee M, Miclau T, Hu D, Werb Z, Helms J: The role of angiogenesis in bone regeneration. 46th Annual Meeting of the Orthopedic Research Society, Orlando, 2000.

Acta Hæmatologica

Acta Haematol 2001;106:157–161

Role of Hematopoietic Growth Factors in Angiogenesis

Domenico Ribatti[a] Angelo Vacca[b] Giuseppe De Falco[b] Roberto Ria[b] Luisa Roncali[a] Franco Dammacco[b]

[a]Department of Human Anatomy and Histology, and [b]Department of Biomedical Sciences and Human Oncology, University of Bari Medical School, Bari, Italy

Key Words
Angiogenesis · Antiangiogenesis · Growth factors · Hematological malignancies · Hematopoiesis

Abstract
In early ontogeny, hematopoiesis is closely associated with angiogenesis. This article reviews recent studies of the effect of hematopoietic growth factors on several endothelial cell functions together with recent findings about angiogenesis and antiangiogenic therapies in hematopoietic malignancies such as leukemia, lymphoma and myeloma.

Early Development of the Endothelial and Hematopoietic Lineages Is Closely Linked Spatially

The relationship between endothelial cells (EC) and hematopoietic cells (HC) has been seen as an indication that a common progenitor, the hemangioblast, gives rise to both cell types in the yolk sac blood islands, i.e. the initial site of hematopoiesis and blood vessel formation during mammalian development [1]. These blood islands derive from aggregates of mesodermal cells that colonize the presumptive yolk sac. The central cells within these aggregates give rise to the embryonic HC while the peripheral populations (angioblasts) differentiate to EC which form the first vascular structures that surround the inner blood cells.

Evidence for the existence of the hemangioblast comes from observations that angiogenic and hematopoietic precursors express some common molecular epitopes. Single embryonic stem cells in culture express the vascular endothelial growth factor receptor-2 (VEGFR-2) and give rise to clones containing hematopoietic progenitors, committed angioblasts, or both cell types [2]. VEGFR-2 knockout mice lack yolk sac blood vessels and organized blood vessels and show a severe reduction in hematopoietic progenitors [2]. It has been demonstrated that VEGFR-2+ mesodermal cells isolated from the posterior area of presomitic chick embryos can differentiate into VEGFR-2+ EC or VEGFR-2– HC, when cultured in vitro in the presence or absence of VEGF, respectively [2]. These data suggest that VEGF is involved in hematopoiesis through angiogenesis.

HC and EC share the expression of genes such as CD34, erythropoietin receptor (EpoR), VEGFR-1, VEGFR-2, GATA-2, PECAM-1, SCL/TAL-1 and Tie-2 [3, 4]. Recent work has suggested that SCL/TAL-1 and VEGFR-2 are coexpressed in isolated mesodermal cells that give rise to EC. Conversely, HC seem to express SCL/

KARGER
Fax + 41 61 306 12 34
E-Mail karger@karger.ch
www.karger.com

0001–5792/01/1064–0157$17.50/0

Accessible online at:
www.karger.com/journals/aha

Prof. Domenico Ribatti, MD
Department of Human Anatomy and Histology
Policlinico, Piazza Giulio Cesare, 11
I–70124 Bari (Italy)
Tel. +39 080 547 82 40, Fax +39 080 547 83 10, E-Mail ribatti@anatomia.uniba.it

TAL-1 and not VEGFR-2. The maturation of blood vessels implies a sequential pattern of expression in which SCL/TAL-1 and VEGFR-2 are expressed first, followed by PECAM-1, CD34, VE-cadherin and later Tie-2. Finally, the SCL/TAL-1 expression is downregulated in mature vessel EC.

Development of HC

Hematopoiesis involves the proliferation and differentiation of hematopoietic stem cells (HSC) to yield erythroid, myeloid and lymphoid lineages. Hematopoiesis prior to the formation of the fetal liver is known as 'primitive hematopoiesis' and is distinguished from adult-type definitive hematopoiesis by the specific expression of embryonic-type globin in nucleated erythrocytes.

Although primitive hematopoiesis and committed hematopoiesis progenitors can be detected in the mouse yolk sac as early as 7–8.5 days postcoitum, neither the colony-forming units in the spleen nor long-term repopulating HSC are present in the yolk sac before circulation [3, 4]. In the mouse embryo, a preliver intraembryonic site of potent definitive hematopoiesis has been identified in an axial mesodermal region, called either the para-aortic splanchnopleural mesoderm region (8.5–9.5 days postcoitum) or the aorta-gonad-mesonephros (thereafter) containing the dorsal aorta, genital ridge/gonads, and pro-/mesonephros [5].

Before circulation is established, progenitors emerging in the intraembryonic mesoderm are capable of generating all hematopoietic lineages. In contrast, yolk sac progenitors have a restricted proliferative capacity and predominantly differentiate into erythroid cells and occasionally into monocytes and megakaryocytes. After the establishment of circulation, multipotent cells in the blood vessels colonize the hemopoietic rudiments. In birds, the first aspect of intraembryonic hematopoiesis is prominent during embryonic day 3 as endothelium-associated 'intra-aortic clusters' [6]. Between day 6 and 8, diffuse hematopoiesis then occurs as 'para-aortic foci' not associated with endothelium in the dorsal mesentery ventral to the aorta [6].

It has been reported that transient contact with endoderm or ectoderm changes the behavior of primitive mesodermal cells and that this effect is mimicked by treatment with several cytokines, namely VEGF, fibroblast growth factor-2 (FGF-2), transforming growth factor-β1 (TGF-β1) and epidermal growth factor (EGF) [7]. Primitive endoderm might be the source of signals that guide primitive mesodermal cells toward an EC fate, since angioblasts arise specifically from splanchnopleural (endoderm-associated) but not splanchnopleural (ectoderm-associated) lateral mesoderm. Hematopoietic organ rudiments formed of mesoderm and endoderm, such as the thymus and liver, do not give rise to hematopoietic progenitors, but require colonization by extrinsic progenitors. The absence of hematopoiesis in organ cultures of both rudiments, isolated early in ontogeny, showed that HC cell generation does not occur in situ. This is also true of the bone marrow, the main hematopoietic organ in adult mammals, which is thought to be colonized by stem cells of fetal liver origin.

HSC Markers

CD34+ HSC are detected at low numbers in bone marrow, fetal liver, and umbilical cord blood [8] and express the newly discovered early HSC marker AC133 [9]. Human-derived AC133+ cells are able to repopulate sheep bone marrow and can thus be considered pluripotent HSC. Expression of CD34 and AC133 diminishes with maturation and differentiation when all terminally differentiated HC fail to express AC133 [9].

Role of HSC in Angiogenesis

HSCs play an important role in angiogenesis during embryogenesis. AML-1 mutant embryos, which lack definitive hematopoiesis, did not generate definitive HSCs and exhibited defective vasculature in the head and pericardium [10]. Vascular phenotypes in AML-1 mutants, such as poor branching of the cardinal vein in the head and poor network formation in the pericardium, are quite similar to those observed in angiopoietin-1 (Ang-1) mutant embryos. Furthermore, migration of ECs in AML-1-mutant embryos is severely disorganized. Disrupted angiogenesis was rescued by the addition of HSC or Ang-1. AML-1 is expressed in EC in sites where early HSC are thought to emerge, such as the yolk sac, vitelline and umbilical arteries, and the aorta-gonad-mesonephros region.

CD34+ HSC stimulated with hematopoietic growth factors [such as kit ligand, interleukin-3 (IL-3), granulocyte-macrophage colony-stimulating factor (GM-CSF) and granulocyte colony-stimulating factor (G-CSF)] release VEGF which, in turn, plays a role in progenitor cell proliferation and trafficking, increasing the release of hematopoietic growth factors by bone marrow EC and augmenting the chemokine-induced transendothelial progenitor cell migration. Similarly, megakaryocytes, stimulated with hematopoietic growth factors, such as IL-3 and thrombopoietin, release VEGF [11]. The consequent increased proliferation of microvessels in close contact with megakaryocytes could be important for efficient platelet production and increased vascular permeability, and endothelial fenestration induced by VEGF could contribute to platelet release.

Role of Hematopoietic Cytokines in Angiogenesis

Hematopoiesis is regulated by several cytokines and ILs including G-CSF, GM-CSF, IL-3, IL-4, IL-6 and IL-8. These molecules, formerly regarded as specific for the hematopoietic system, also affect certain EC functions [3, 4, 12, 13].

Receptors for G-CSF and GM-CSF have been detected on the surface of EC. These cytokines induce EC to migrate and proliferate and are angiogenic in vivo in the rabbit cornea. GM-CSF also induces angiogenesis in rat connective tissue by a direct effect on EC and/or by the recruitment and activation of macrophages that release their own angiogenic factors.

Human EC express receptors for IL-3. IL-4, a lymphocyte growth and differentiation factor, stimulates the growth of EC. IL-6, a B cell differentiation factor, regulates the growth of vascular cells and its overexpression in the central nervous system of transfecting mice correlates with neovascularization. IL-6 mRNA is expressed in EC during the angiogenesis that accompanies folliculogenesis and formation of decidua. Furthermore, IL-6 participates in an autocrine manner in the growth of Kaposi's sarcoma, and exerts an autocrine activity in middle T antigen-transformed EC. It is also secreted by non-Hodgkin's lymphoma, lymphoblastic leukemia and multiple myeloma, tumors in which the extent of angiogenesis is related to neoplastic progression. Viral IL-6-positive mice displayed increased hematopoiesis in the myeloid, erythroid and megakaryocytic lineages and gave rise to highly vascularized tumors. Finally, IL-8, which regulates the functions of mature myeloid cells, is an angiogenic factor that induces proliferation and chemotaxis of human EC.

EC from some sources express EpoR. Epo induces EC proliferation and migration, and has been shown to stimulate angiogenesis on rat aortic rings in vitro [14].

We have demonstrated that recombinant human Epo (rHuEpo) induces a proangiogenic phenotype in human EC [15]. This phenotype included both early (i.e. increase in cell proliferation and MMP-2 production) and late angiogenic events (differentiation into vascular tubes). Accordingly, EC expressed EpoR that bound to JAK-2 and induced its transient activation after rHuEpo exposure. In the CAM assay, the angiogenic activity of the rHuEpo was quantitatively and qualitatively similar to that exerted by the angiogenic cytokine FGF-2 in the absence of a significant mononuclear cell infiltrate, and EC of the CAM expressed EpoR that colocalizes with factor VIII positivity. Taken together, these data demonstrate that Epo acts as a direct angiogenic factor.

In a recently described in vitro model for human bone marrow angiogenesis, in which pericytes and basal lamina matrix were associated with EC and formed fully organized capillary tubes [16], the addition of Epo, stem cell factor, GM-CSF or G-CSF, induced a highly significant increase in tube formation. When Epo and G-CSF were added, this increase was larger than the maximum increase observed with VEGF.

The Malignant Counterparts

In several cancers of hematopoietic lineage, including non-Hodgkin's lymphoma, lymphoblastic leukemia, B cell chronic lymphocytic leukemia, acute myeloid leukemia and multiple myeloma, neoplastic progression is clearly related to the degree of angiogenesis [17].

In B cell non-Hodgkin's lymphoma, an increase in microvessel density in lymph nodes correlates with the severity of the disease. Increased density has also been reported in bone marrow of active multiple myeloma in comparison with nonactive multiple myeloma and monoclonal gammopathy of undetermined significance [18]. Patients with active myeloma have elevated levels of angiogenic cytokines such as FGF-2 and VEGF, as well as increased bone marrow levels of mast cells which secrete a variety of angiogenic factors, all playing a role both in tumor cell growth and survival, as well as in bone marrow angiogenesis. Furthermore, in myeloma, neovascularization, plasma cell angiogenic potential and matrix metalloproteinase-2 secretion parallel disease progression.

Additional studies illustrate the increased bone marrow angiogenesis in both lymphoid and myeloid leukemias [19, 20]. Leukemias originate from HSC at different stages of their maturation and differentiation. It is now well established that acute leukemias originate from immature HSC that can undergo self-renewal, whereas less aggressive leukemias such as chronic leukemias seem to originate from the more mature committed HSC.

Similar to cytokine-stimulated HSC, the malignant counterparts of early HC, such as blasts of acute leukemia, constitutively release VEGF [21]. In acute leukemia, overexpression of VEGF in the bone marrow microenvironment may result in a permanent increase in vascular permeability and fenestration, contributing to release of the leukemic cells into the circulation. One might speculate that malignant transformation results in sustained upregulation of the regulatory pathways also involved in cytokine-induced production of VEGF by normal proliferating progenitors. Further studies also suggest that the release of VEGF in acute leukemia results in increased vascular density in the bone marrow, which may indirectly support the growth of the malignant cells similar to solid tumors, and is associated with poor outcome. It has been demonstrated that B cell chronic lymphocytic leukemia express VEGF mRNA and produce VEGF protein. Moreover, VEGF produced by chronic lymphocytic leukemia cells stimulates EC proliferation and in vivo angiogenesis.

EC exposed to recombinant human VEGF manifested an increased mRNA for several hematopoietic growth factors including G-CSF, GM-CSF, stem cell factor and IL-6 which, in turn, may act as growth factors for myeloid and lymphoid malignant cells, suggesting that VEGF may play a role in the growth of hematopoietic neoplasms via a paracrine mechanism. In multiple myeloma, stimulation of IL-6 secretion by marrow stromal cells was previously shown for tumor necrosis factor-α (TNF-α), IL-1 and TGF-β, but had not been described for angiogenic cytokines. It has recently been demonstrated that VEGF is a paracrine mediator supporting myeloma cell growth through the induction of IL-6 release by bone marrow stroma [22]. Furthermore, elevated levels of FGF-2 were detected in urine from patients with acute lymphoblastic leukemia and lymphoma [17], and in children with acute lymphoblastic leukemia, elevated levels of FGF-2 in the urine were associated with increased bone marrow vessel density [17].

Therapeutic Possibilities

Antiangiogenesis was proposed as a cancer therapy over 20 years ago and the list of compounds reported to possess antiangiogenic activity is extensive. Clinical trials of potential inhibitors, however, are very recent. Inhibitors are grouped as class 1 (specific and semispecific) and class 2 (nonspecific), depending on whether they inhibit proliferation and/or migration of EC only, or are also cytotoxic for tumor cells. Antiangiogenic therapy may be applicable to a wide variety of solid tumors and there is evidence that tumors do not develop resistance to the effects of antiangiogenic agents, which is most likely attributable to the low mutagenic potential of EC [23].

Thalidomide was originally used in Europe for the treatment of morning sickness in the 1950s but withdrawn from the market in the 1960s because of reports of teratogenicity and phocomelia associated with its use. The renewed interest in thalidomide stems from its broad spectrum of pharmacologic and immunologic effects. It has powerful antiangiogenic activity and can eradicate experimental tumors in mice. The discovery that thalidomide inhibits angiogenesis led to preclinical and phase I/II trials of thalidomide as an anticancer agent in solid tumors and hematological malignancies [24]. In a clinical trial comprising 84 chemotherapy-refractory, multiple myeloma patients, it induced a marked and durable response in approximately one third, as shown by the reduction of at least 25% of the M-component. The study considered a gradual increase in the dose of thalidomide up to a maximum daily dose of 800 mg. Thalidomide also seems to be effective in myelodysplastic syndromes, myeloproliferative disorders, acute myelogenous leukemia and myelofibrosis.

Conventional cytotoxic chemotherapeutic drugs have been used at low (nanomolar) and noncytotoxic concentrations as an antiangiogenic [25]. Antiendothelial effects have been demonstrated in vitro for cyclophosphamide, 5-fluorouracil, and mitomycin C, and short-term antiangiogenic effects have been demonstrated in vivo for vincristine, vinblastine, doxorubicin, mitaxantrone, etoposide, paclitaxel, 6-methylmercaptopurine, tegafur, 9-amino-20(s)-camptothecin, topotecan, camptosan and combrestatin. The presence of dividing EC in newly forming tumor blood vessels should render such vessels – in contrast to their mature, quiescent counterparts found in normal adult tissues – sensitive to the cytotoxic effects of such drugs in a manner similar to dividing bone marrow cells [26]. In this context, it has been demonstrated in murine models of leukemia that low-dose cyclophosphamide, used as an antiangiogenic drug, may avoid drug resistance and eradicate established disease 3-fold more effectively than the conventional maximum-tolerable dose [26].

Blocking the interaction of VEGF with its receptors has been shown to be another option for antiangiogenic treatment [24]. Antibodies to VEGF or expression of a dominant-negative VEGF receptor inhibit tumor growth in vivo without affecting tumor cell proliferation. In animals treated with anti-VEGF antibodies, the density of blood vessels in tumor sections is lower than in the tumors of control animals, showing that the inhibitory effect of the antibody on tumor growth is mediated by a blockage of the angiogenic activity of VEGF. By using a neutralizing monoclonal antibody specific for human VEGFR-2, it has been demonstrated that inhibition of VEGFR-2 either in vitro or in vivo blocked proliferation of VEGFR-2+ human leukemias, and it has been suggested that blocking VEGFR-2 signaling may represent a novel therapeutic approach to the treatment of a subset of acute leukemias.

These findings have provided a rationale for the use of antiangiogenic drugs in the treatment of hematological malignancies that are suboptimally treated with cytotoxic therapy.

Acknowledgements

This work was supported in part by grants from the Associazione Italiana per la Lotta al Neuroblastoma, Genoa; Associazione Italiana per la Ricerca sul Cancro, Milan; Ministero dell'Università e della Ricerca Scientifica e Tecnologica (Cofinanziamento 1999 'Multiple Myeloma: New Biological Insights Assay and Their Therapeutic Implications'). We apologize for not having been able to cite many important papers because of the editorial policy of limiting the length of the reference list.

References

1 Murray PDF: The development in vitro of blood of the chick embryo. Proc R Soc B 1934; 111:497–524.
2 Yancopoulos GD, Davis S, Gale NW, Rudge JS, Wiehand SJ, Holash HW, Holash HJ: Vascular-specific growth factor and blood vessel formation. Nature 2000;407:242–248.
3 Ribatti D, Vacca A, Roncali L, Dammacco F: Hematopoiesis and angiogenesis: A link between two apparently independent processes. J Hematother Stem Cell Res 2000;9:13–19.
4 Suda T, Takakura N, Oike Y: Hematopoiesis and angiogenesis. Int J Hematol 2000;71:99–107.
5 Delassus S, Titley I, Enver T: Functional and molecular analysis of hematopoietic progenitors derived from the aorta-gonad-mesonephros region of the mouse embryo. Blood 1999; 94:1495–1503.
6 Jaffredo T, Gautier R, Brajeul V, Dieterlen-Lievre F: Tracing the progeny of the aortic hemangioblast in the avian embryo. Dev Biol 2000;224:204–214.
7 Pardanaud L, Dieterlen-Lievre F: Manipulation of the angiopoietic/hematopoietic commitment in the avian embryo. Development 1999;126:617–627.
8 Goodell MA: $CD34^+$ or $CD34^-$: Does it really matter? Blood 1999;94:2545–2547.
9 Gehling UM, Ergun S, Schumacher U, Wagener C, Pantel K, Otte M, Schuch G, Schafhausen P, Mende T, Kilic N, Kuge K, Schafer B, Hossfeld DK, Fiedler W: In vitro differentiation of endothelial cells from Ac133-positive progenitor cells. Blood 2000;95:3106–3112.
10 Takakura N, Waranabe T, Svenobu S, Yamada Y, Noda T, Ito Y, Satake M, Suda A: Role for hematopoietic stem cells in promoting angiogenesis. Cell 2000;102:199–209.
11 Mohle R, Green D, Moore MAS, Nachman RL, Rafii S: Constitutive production and thrombin-induced release of vascular endothelial growth factor by human megakaryocytes and platelet. Proc Natl Acad Sci USA 1997;94: 633–637.
12 Bussolino F, Bocchietto E, Silvagno F, Soldi R, Arese M, Mantovani A: Actions of molecules which regulate hemopoiesis on endothelial cells: Memoirs of common ancestors? Pathol Res Pract 1994;190:834–839.
13 Bikfalvi A, Hanz ZC: Angiogenic factors are hematopoietic factors and vice versa. Leukemia 1994;8:523–529.
14 Carlini RG, Reyes AA, Rothstein M: Recombinant human erythropoietin stimulates angiogenesis in vitro. Kidney Int 1995;47:740–745.
15 Ribatti D, Presta M, Vacca A, Ria R, Giuliani R, Dell'Era P, Nico B, Roncali L, Dammacco F: Human erythropoietin induces a pro-angiogenic phenotype in cultured endothelial cells and stimulates neovascularization in vivo. Blood 1999;93:2627–2636.
16 Pelletier L, Regnard J, Fellmann D, Chabord P: An in vitro model for the study of human bone marrow angiogenesis: Role of hematopoietic cytokine. Lab Invest 2000;80:501–511.
17 Bertolini F, Mancuso P, Gobbi A, Pruneri G: The thin red line: Angiogenesis in normal and malignant hematopoiesis. Exp Hematol 2000; 28:993–1000.
18 Vacca A, Ribatti D, Presta M, Minischetti M, Iurlaro M, Ria R, Albini A, Bussolino F, Dammacco F: Bone marrow neovascularization, plasma cell angiogenic potential, and matrix metalloproteinase-2 secretion parallel progression of human multiple myeloma. Blood 1999; 93:3064–3073.
19 Perez-Atayade AR, Sallan SE, Tedrow U, Connors S, Allred E, Folkman J: Spectrum of tumor angiogenesis in the bone marrow of children with acute lymphoblastic leukemia. Am J Pathol 1997;150:815–821.
20 Padro T, Ruiz S, Bieker R, Burger H, Steins M, Kieast J, Buchner T, Berdel WE, Mesters RM: Increased angiogenesis in the bone marrow of patients with acute myeloid leukemia. Blood 2000;95:2637–2644.
21 Dias S, Hattori K, Zhu Z, Heissig B, Choy M, Lane W, Wu Y, Chadburn A, Hyjek E, Gill M, Hicklin DJ, Moore MAS, Rafii S: Autocrine stimulation of VEGFR-2 activated human leukemic cell growth and migration. J Clin Invest 2000;106:511–521.
22 Dankbar B, Padro T, Leo R, Feldmann B, Kropff M, Mesters RM, Serve H, Berdel WE, Kienast J: Vascular endothelial growth factor and interleukin-6 in paracrine tumor-stromal cell interactions in multiple myeloma. Blood 2000;95:2630–2636.
23 Talks KL, Harris AL: Current status of antiangiogenic factors. Br J Haematol 2000;109:477–489.
24 Anderson KC: Thalidomide: Therapeutic potential in hematologic malignancies. Semin Hematol 2000;37(suppl 3):1–4.
25 Vacca A, Iurlaro M, Ribatti D, Minischetti M, Nico B, Ria R, Pellegrino A, Dammacco F: Antiangiogenesis is produced by nontoxic doses of vinblastine. Blood 1999;94:4143–4155.
26 Kerbel KS, Viloria-Petit A, Klement G, Rak J: 'Accidental' anti-angiogenic drugs: Anti-oncogene directed signal transduction inhibitors and conventional chemotherapeutic agents as examples. Eur J Cancer 2000;36:1248–1257.

Acta Hæmatologica

Acta Haematol 2001;106:162–169

Bone Marrow Angiogenesis and Plasma Cell Angiogenic and Invasive Potential in Patients with Active Multiple Myeloma

Angelo Vacca[a] Domenico Ribatti[b] Aldo M. Roccaro[a] Roberto Ria[a] Loredana Palermo[a] Franco Dammacco[a]

[a]Department of Biomedical Sciences and Human Oncology, and [b]Department of Human Anatomy and Histology, University of Bari Medical School, Bari, Italy

Key Words
Angiogenesis · Endothelial cell · Invasion · Metalloproteinases · Multiple myeloma · Tumor progression

Abstract
Factor VIII-related antigen-positive microvessel areas were measured by both immunohistochemistry and computerized image analysis in patients with active multiple myeloma (MM), nonactive MM and monoclonal gammopathies of undetermined significance (MGUS). A 5- to 6-fold larger area was found in patients with active MM compared to the other two groups. The conditioned medium (CM) of their bone marrow plasma cells stimulated endothelial cell proliferation and chemotaxis, monocyte chemotaxis and angiogenesis in vivo [chick embryo chorioallantoic membrane (CAM) system] more strongly and frequently than the CM of patients with nonactive MM and MGUS. An immunoassay of plasma cell lysates gave significantly higher levels of fibroblast growth factor-2 (FGF-2) in patients with active MM than in the other two groups, and a neutralizing anti-FGF-2 antibody inhibited by 54–68% the biological activity exerted by the CM in vitro and in the CAM. In situ hybridization of bone marrow plasma cells and gelatin zymography of CM showed that patients with active MM express higher levels of matrix metalloproteinase-2 (MMP-2) mRNA and protein than those with nonactive MM and MGUS, whereas MMP-9 expression and secretion overlapped in all groups. Overall data suggest that patients with active MM represent the vascular phase of plasma cell tumors that is triggered by bone marrow plasma cells, at least partly, through FGF-2 and MMP-2. Both angiogenesis and MMP-2 secretion can account for intramedullary and extramedullary spreading of plasma cells during the active MM.

Introduction

Angiogenesis occurs during embryo development and in postnatal life in wound repair and cyclically in the female genital system [1]. It is limited in time and the result of an equilibrium between activator and inhibitor systems that together keep the microcirculation in a quiescent state with very low proliferation and turnover of the endothelial cells (EC). These cells rest on a specialized form of the extracellular matrix, the basement membrane [2]. Angiogenesis develops through [3] (1) basement membrane degradation by the proteolytic enzymes, including metalloproteinases (MMPs), secreted by the EC, which results in the formation of tiny sprouts penetrating into

KARGER
Fax + 41 61 306 12 34
E-Mail karger@karger.ch
www.karger.com

0001–5792/01/1064–0162$17.50/0

Accessible online at:
www.karger.com/journals/aha

Prof. Angelo Vacca, MD
Department of Biomedical Sciences and Human Oncology
Section of Internal Medicine and Clinical Oncology, Policlinico
Piazza Giulio Cesare, 11, I–70124 Bari (Italy)
Tel. +39 080 559 31 06, Fax +39 080 547 88 20, E-Mail avacca@hotmail.com

the stroma; (2) migration towards the angiogenic stimulus of EC below the sprout; (3) canalization, branching and formation of a functional vascular plexus, and (4) perivascular apposition of pericytes and synthesis of basement membrane constituents by both EC and pericytes.

Tumor angiogenesis develops through the same steps, but is unlimited in time, and characterized by a 30- to 40-fold proliferative activity of EC [1]. It is essential for tumor progression, in terms of growth, invasion and metastasis. The progression from in situ to invasive and metastatic solid tumors is accompanied by the transition from avascular to the vascular phase [4].

Bone Marrow Angiogenesis in Multiple Myeloma Parallels Disease Progression

Bone marrow biopsies of patients with active multiple myeloma (MM; diagnosis, relapse, leukemic progression), nonactive MM (complete/objective response or off-treatment plateau phase) and with monoclonal gammopathies of undetermined significance (MGUS) were investigated for microvessel density [5]. Six-micrometer deparaffinized and hydrated sections were sequentially incubated with a monoclonal (murine) antibody to the EC marker factor VIII-related antigen, a biotin-labeled (horse) anti-mouse IgG and avidin-peroxidase conjugate, then stained red with a 3-amino-9-ethylcarbazole solution and counterstained with hematoxylin. Among all the stained vessels, microvessels (e.g. capillaries and small venules) were identified on 250× fields within a superimposed 484-point square reticle of 12.5×10^{-2} mm^2: the area they occupied ('microvessel area') was calculated by using the planimetric method of 'point counting', according to which the area equaled the sum of points that hit microvessels. The microvessel area was normalized to the cellular area (reticle area minus dense connective tissue, bone lamellae, fat, necrosis and hemorrhagic areas) by using a computerized image analysis system (KS-300, Zeiss). The very few megakaryocytes also stained with the factor VIII-related antigen were easily distinguishable from microvessels by their morphology.

Figure 1 shows that the microvessel area of patients with active MM was 5- to 6-fold wider (as average value) than that of patients with nonactive MM and with MGUS. The widest area was associated with rapidly progressive disease. The area of patients with nonactive MM differed only marginally from that of patients with MGUS.

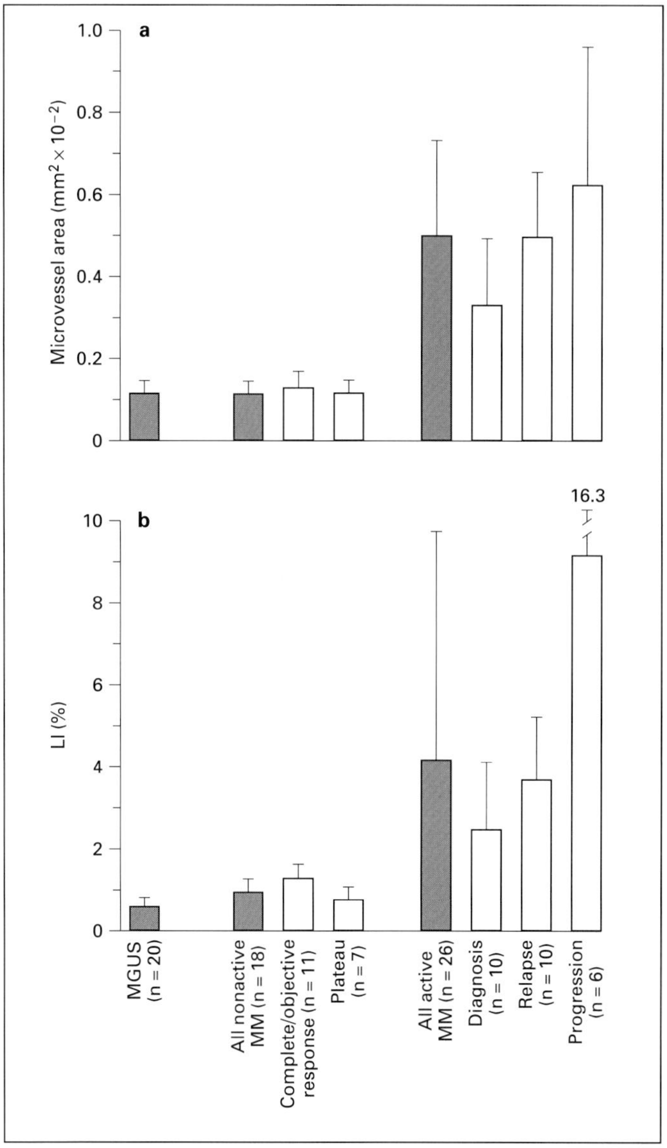

Fig. 1. Symmetric changes of microvessel area (**a**) and plasma cell LI (**b**) in the bone marrow of patients. The microvessel area and LI were significantly correlated (R^2 = 0.73–0.94; $p < 0.01$). Number of patients is given in parentheses.

Figure 1 also shows that the area was strictly correlated with the plasma cell proliferative activity, as evaluated by the labeling index (LI%) technique [6]. Therefore, the angiogenesis is denser, the faster the plasma cell proliferation is, suggesting that angiogenesis favors the expansion of the MM cell mass.

The differences in microvessel area between patients with active MM and other patient groups are also shown in figure 2. Figure 2 shows that microvessels in patients

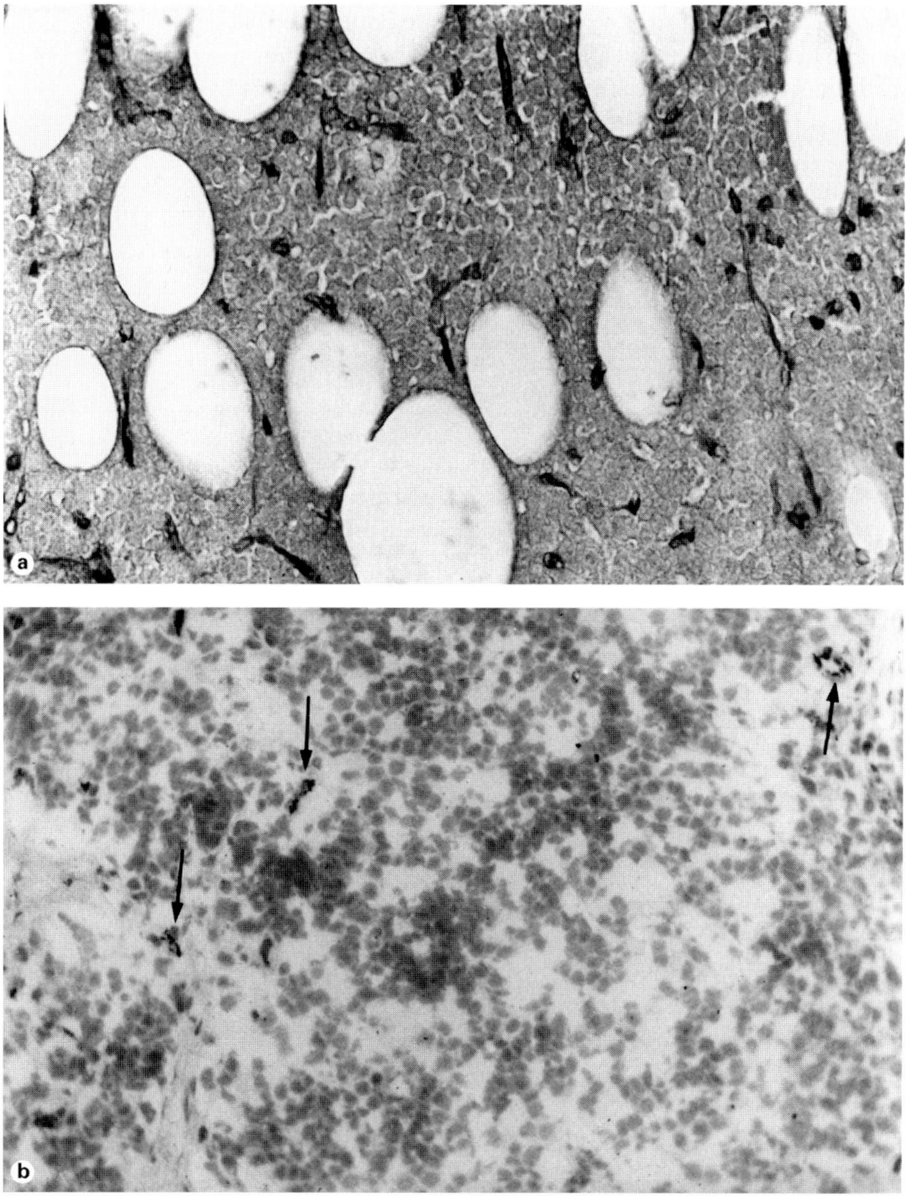

Fig. 2. The two opposite conditions in the bone marrow. **a** Numerous, thin, winding microvessels, some of which as clustered EC, in a patient with active MM (relapse). **b** Very few microvessels (arrows) in a patient with nonactive MM (plateau phase).

with active MM were thin, winding, often without visible lumina and characterized by single or clustered EC and small endothelial 'sprouts' without lumen, in contrast to straight vessels without sprouts in patients with nonactive MM and MGUS. As the progression from in situ to invasive and metastatic solid tumors is accompanied and enhanced by the switch from the prevascular to the vascular phase, these in situ findings suggest that the active MM may represent the 'vascular phase' of plasma cell tumors, and nonactive MM and MGUS their 'prevascular phase'. Bone marrow angiogenesis may therefore favor progression from MGUS or nonactive MM to active MM.

Myeloma Plasma Cells of Active MM Patients May Trigger the Vascular Phase

The association between Kaposi's sarcoma and MM, however rare, has been described [7], and the angiogenic ability of MM plasma cells has been tentatively suggested [8]. In our study, the presence of bone marrow angiogenesis in patients with active MM prompted us to investigate whether their plasma cells, harvested in close proximity to the biopsy site, do possess an angiogenic capacity, i.e. whether they are capable of inducing an angiogenic phenotype in cultured human EC and angiogenesis in vivo.

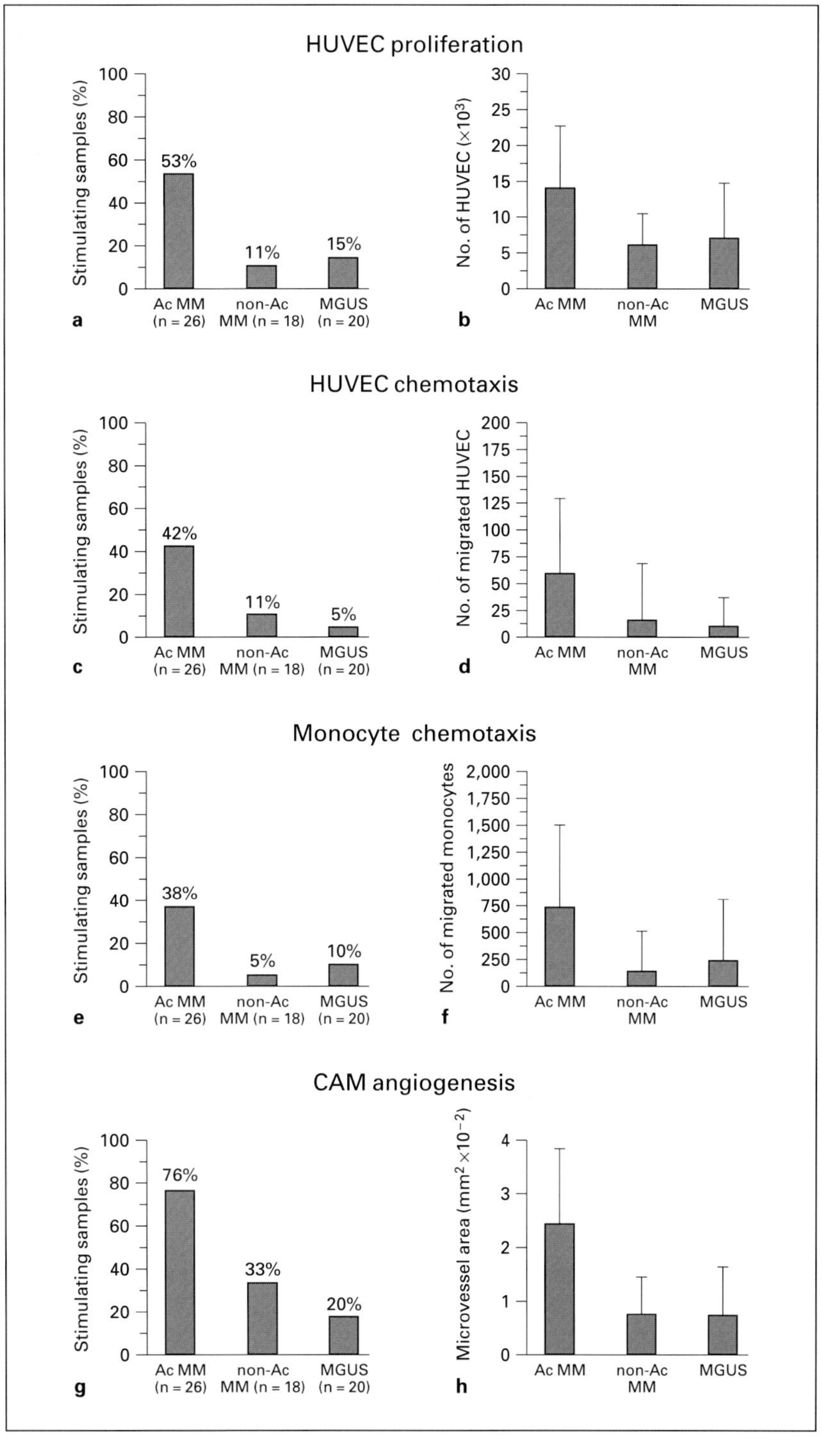

Fig. 3. Effect of CM of bone marrow plasma cells from patients with active MM (Ac MM), nonactive MM (non-Ac MM) and MGUS on HUVEC proliferation, chemotaxis and human monocyte chemotaxis, as well as on the chick embryo CAM angiogenesis.

Bone marrow aspirates were subjected to plasma cell enrichment through [9]: (1) Ficoll-Hypaque density gradient centrifugation; (2) removal of T cells (by E-rosetting), monocytes and fibroblasts (by plastic adhesion); (3) subtraction of plasma cells by magnetic microbeads coated with an antibody to the plasma cell marker CD38, and (4) bead detachment in a 12-hour culture. Enriched plasma cells, consisting of >95% tumor plasma cells and their clonally related cells, were cultured for 24 h in serum-free RPMI 1640 containing 1% glutamine. This medium was then collected, centrifuged sequentially at 1,200 and 12,000 rpm, respectively, for 10 min, filtered through sterilized 0.22-μm pore-size filters and stored at −80°C 'conditioned medium' (CM). The CM was tested for its ability to induce the EC functions needed for angiogenesis to develop, such as proliferation and chemotaxis and for monocyte chemotaxis that implies cell activation and consequent secretion of angiogenic factors and EMC-degrading enzymes [10].

Human umbilical vein EC (HUVEC) at the second passage were exposed on days 0, 2 and 4 to complete medium (positive control) and serum-free (starvation) medium (negative control), to which 1:1 (vol:vol) CM was added, and were counted by a colorimetric method on day 6. Figure 3a shows that 14 out of 26 (53%) CM from active MM patients stimulated HUVEC proliferation, as against only 2 out of 18 (11%) CM from nonactive MM patients and 3 out of 20 (15%) CM from MGUS patients. Figure 3b also shows that proliferation was higher when cells were exposed to the CM of active MM patients.

HUVEC were also induced to migrate in response to the plasma cell CM. By using the Boyden chamber technique, HUVEC were seeded in the upper compartment of the chamber and the CM in the lower compartment, which was separated from the former by a 12-μm pore-size polycarbonate gelatin-coated filter. After being incubated for 6 h, the cells that had migrated to the lower side of the filter were stained and counted. Figure 3c shows that a higher proportion of CM from active MM patients stimulated HUVEC chemotaxis, and figure 3d that the stimulation induced by such CM was stronger. The monocyte chemotaxis stimulation test was carried out in a similar manner. Again, figure 3e and f shows that the CM of patients with active MM gave results similar to those described for HUVEC chemotaxis.

To stimulate angiogenesis in vivo, we used the chick embryo chorioallantoic membrane (CAM) sponge system [11]. The CAMs were examined daily until day 12 (when the angiogenic response peaks) by a stereomicroscope (Zeiss). On day 12, the sponges and the underlying and immediately adjacent CAM portions were removed, embedded in paraffin, sectioned, routinely stained and processed on 250× fields for the microvessel area by using the planimetric method applied to bone marrow biopsies. The CM of 20 out of 26 (76%) active MM patients induced an angiogenic response that presented as a dense capillary growth with numerous capillaries converging towards the sponge like many spokes. By contrast, only 33 and 20% of CM from nonactive MM and MGUS patients, respectively, did induce the response. Moreover, the extent of the microvessel area was larger in the sponges loaded with the CM of active MM patients. The values of the bone marrow and CAM-sponge microvessel areas were compared for each patient, showing that both areas were significantly correlated ($r = 0.81$, $p < 0.001$).

The Angiogenic Ability of Plasma Cells Is Mediated by Fibroblast Growth Factor-2 and Other Angiogenic Factors

We obtained evidence in favor of fibroblast growth factor-2 (FGF-2) production by MM plasma cells during the active phase of the disease [9]. Cell lysates obtained from constant amounts of enriched plasma cells ($2–3 \times 10^6$) for each patient were analyzed for FGF-2 levels by means of the ELISA. We showed that the FGF-2 levels were significantly ($p < 0.01$) higher in the lysates of active MM patients (153 ± 59 pg FGF-2/100 μg protein) compared with those of nonactive MM and MGUS patients (23 ± 17 and 31 ± 18, respectively). These results agree with those obtained in patients with B-cell chronic lymphocytic leukemia, showing that intracellular expression of FGF-2 is correlated with disease progression [12].

Based on this finding, we wondered whether FGF-2 was operative, e.g. whether it was actually involved in the in vitro induction of angiogenic phenotype of HUVEC and angiogenesis in the CAM by the plasma cell CM. We therefore tried to find out whether inhibition of FGF-2 by means of a specific antibody also meant inhibition of the CM angiogenic capacity. To that effect, we analyzed 7 CM of active MM patients that induced both HUVEC and monocyte functions in vitro and angiogenesis in the CAM. The addition of a polyclonal anti-FGF-2 antibody (kindly provided by Prof. M. Presta, University of Brescia, Italy) to the CM (400 mg/ml) inhibited the CM-induced HUVEC proliferation and chemotaxis, monocyte chemotaxis and CAM angiogenesis by 46–68%. Hence, the antibody did not produce complete, but only partial inhibition. In addition, there was no correlation between FGF-2 plasma cell levels and extent of the bone marrow microvessel area (data not shown). Both findings suggest that FGF-2 is not the only plasma cell factor capable of inducing bone marrow angiogenesis in MM.

Indeed, hepatocyte growth factor/scatter factor is yet another angiogenic factor that was identified in the CM of both human MM cell lines [13] and in freshly isolated MM cells [14]. Serum levels of this factor are high in 43% of patients at diagnosis, then decline down to normal levels as the response to induction therapy is achieved, though this does not occur if the therapy is ineffective; the levels become high again upon relapse [15]. Based on this observations and also on the fact that the corresponding levels fluctuate concordantly with the M-component serum/urine levels, hepatocyte growth factor/scatter factor was interpreted as a typical secretion product of MM plasma cells. In addition, vascular endothelial cell growth factor is produced by MM plasma cells and may be involved in the stimulation of angiogenesis, as well as in autocrine and paracrine loops of plasma cell growth [16].

Still other factors may be responsible for bone marrow angiogenesis in MM: (1) the already demonstrated plasma cell secretion products, such as transforming growth factor-β and IL-1β [17]; the latter factor, however, is only indirectly angiogenic insofar as it stimulates the bone marrow microenvironment cells to secrete IL-6 and the platelets to secrete the platelet-derived growth factor [18] and (2) IL-6, IL-8, G-CSF, GM-CSF, TNF-α [19] secreted by bone marrow microenvironment cells recruited and activated by myeloma plasma cells (via chemokines?, FGF-2?). It is worth noting that IL-6, IL-8, GM-CSF and IL-1β are secreted mostly in the MM-active phase [20] where we found enhanced angiogenesis.

Expression and Secretion of MMP-2 and MMP-9

SB (B cell lymphoblastic leukemia), U266 (MM), CEM and Jurkat (T cell lymphoblastic leukemia) cell lines were evaluated for the expression of MMP-2 and MMP-9 mRNA by in situ hybridization [21]. SB and U266 cells coexpressed the mRNAs. The signal intensity for both mRNAs was similar in the B-lymphoblastic leukemia cell lines SB, while U266 cells showed a more intense MMP-2 mRNA-related signal than that of MMP-9. CEM and Jukart cells expressed MMP-2 mRNA only. The mRNAs were operative, given the fact that the corresponding enzymes were secreted into the CM and detected by sodium dodecyl sulfate-polyacrylamide gel electrophoresis (PAGE) gelatin zymography. MMP-2 and MMP-9 gave rise to gelatinolytic bands with an apparent M_r of 62 and 88 kD, respectively, indicating that both enzymes were present in their cleaved, activated form [22]. According to in situ hybridization pictures, the computerized image analysis of the bands showed that overlapping amounts of MMP-2 and MMP-9 were present in the CM of SB cells, whereas MMP-2 levels were higher than those of MMP-9 in the CM of U266 cells, and the CM of CEM and Jurkat cells contained only MMP-2 gelatinolytic activity. Overall results demonstrate that human lymphoid tumor cells and MM cells constitutively produce significant amounts of the ECM-degrading enzymes MMP-2 and/or MMP-9, which are found in their cleaved, activated form.

Based on these findings, we focused on the invasive potential of bone marrow plasma cells during MM progression [23]. We found that cells of MGUS and MM patients expressed the MMP-2 and MMP-9 mRNA, whereas in cells from control patients (suffering from anemia due to iron or vitamin B_{12} deficiencies) the MMP-2 mRNA was absent or poorly expressed in some instances, as evaluated by in situ hybridization. The MMP-2 mRNA-related signal was stronger in patients with active MM than in those with nonactive MM and with MGUS. The MMP-9 mRNA-related signal was lower than that of MMP-2 in all patient groups and overlapped between the groups.

PAGE gelatin zymography of plasma cell CM showed that plasma cells secrete activated MMP-2 (62-kD form) and lower levels of activated MMP-9 (88-kD form), whereas those from control patients secrete only marginal levels of activated MMP-2. Specifically, quantitation of MMP-2 and MMP-9 by computerized image analysis of the gelatinolytic bands showed that MMP-2 was present in CM of 84% active MM patients at $22.5 \pm 7.4 \times 10^3$ optical density (OD) compared with 27% nonactive MM patients at $12.4 \pm 3.6 \times 10^3$ OD, 25% MGUS patients at $13.4 \pm 5.4 \times 10^3$ OD, and 16% control patients at $4.0 \pm 1.7 \times 10^3$ OD. MMP-9 was cosecreted in 23% active MM patients, 16% nonactive MM patients and 10% MGUS patients. Overall results confirm the findings obtained in the MM cell line U266 and demonstrate that in MM patients MMP-2 is overexpressed and secreted in step with tumor progression.

Given the ability of MMP-2 and MMP-9 to degrade type IV, V, VII and X collagens as well as fibronectin [22], namely the major components of the interstitial stroma and subendothelial basement membrane, the findings suggest that plasma cells of active MM patients are especially capable of invading both the stroma and the basement membrane. Since angiogenesis and major proteolytic activity occur together in close vicinity of plasma cells, conditions of intra- and extramedullary dissemination of these cells are thereby established during active disease.

Involvement of Host Inflammatory Cells

In parallel with enhanced angiogenesis, we have obtained evidence of the increase of mast cell density in the bone marrow of patients with active MM [24]. At the ultrastructural level, the majority of cells displayed semilunar aspects of cytoplasmic granules, suggesting that they were chronically and slowly releasing mediators in response to a degranulatory stimulus.

The study led us to hypothesize that mast cells are recruited and activated in the bone marrow by MM plasma cells, and that angiogenesis is mediated, at least partly, by angiogenic factors contained in their secretory granules. These results are in line with those demonstrating bone marrow angiogenesis in the SCID-hu MM model in close association with a dense stromal cell infiltrate [25]. In other B cell malignancies, such as B cell non-Hodgkin's lymphomas, we found that, similarly to mast cells in MM, macrophage density increases with histological progression, as defined both by Kiel and WF malignancy grades [26]. Overall, our data agree with those showing a close relationship between mast cell/macrophage density and angiogenesis during progression of solid tumors [27].

Possible Prognostic Value of Bone Marrow Angiogenesis in Multiple Myeloma

The prognostic role of angiogenesis has already been demonstrated in patients with solid tumors, including breast, lung, colon, head and neck and prostate carcinoma: increased density of neovessels means poorer prognosis [28]. This relationship is due to the fact that angiogenesis means a greater velocity of growth, and a greater invasive and metastatic capacity of the neoplastic cells. Hence, more vessels mean a locally more advanced and/or already metastatic disease.

We have described that bone marrow angiogenesis in patients with MM and with MGUS is correlated with the proliferating activity of MM plasma cells, rated as LI%. The latter parameter is itself a prognostic factor. Actually, the mean survival is shorter in patients with LI $\geq$ 1% (15 months) than in those with LI <1% (40 months), irrespective of the cell mass [29]. In effect, MM patients with high LI% are still far from the steady state since their mass is in the exponential growth. They respond rapidly to induction cytostatic treatment (the so-called 'early responders'), but their response is short-lived and followed by an equally rapid relapse in connection with massive recruitment into the cell cycle of G0 plasma cells, hence by shorter overall survival [30]. Since LI% refers to the whole MM cell production even small variations (e.g. by 1%) really denote profound changes in the proliferative activity. This must be taken into account when expressing a prognosis. Since we have demonstrated that bone marrow angiogenesis and LI% are closely associated with the various phases in MM activity and are mutually correlated, and since LI% is a prognostic factor, it may well be that the disease in a given state (MGUS, non-active MM) can be supposed to be at risk of progression towards the subsequent larger-mass steady state (active MM) if the bone marrow shows angiogenesis. The risk would be the greater, the larger the microvessel area is, namely it would be 3.9 times as great for each 1% LI increment (by Pearson's r, Spearman's rs and logistic regression analysis). The risk is the same with 0.6% LI increments [6]. Microvessel area variations are therefore less restricted than those of LI% as a risk assessment parameter, and could be a useful guide to prognosis just as LI% is when applied in plasma cell proliferative diseases.

Concluding Remarks

The following conclusions can be drawn from our studies: (1) MGUS and nonactive MM may represent the prevascular phase of plasma cell tumors, and the active MM the vascular phase; (2) tumor plasma cells of active MM patients are able to induce the angiogenic switch via FGF-2 and (3) constitutively express and secrete high levels of MMP-2; (4) bone marrow angiogenesis and MMP-2 (MMP-9) secretion may explain the frequent occurrence of intramedullary and extramedullary localizations in active MM patients; (5) bone marrow angiogenesis defines a risk of progression and may be a prognostic marker, and (6) antiangiogenic (anti-FGF-2) and anti-MMP-2 therapy may have potential clinical applications in active MM patients.

References

1 Carmeliet P: Mechanisms of angiogenesis and arteriogenesis. Nat Med 2000;6:389–395.

2 Bonanno E, Iurlaro M, Madri JA, Nicosia RF: Type IV collagen modulates angiogenesis and neovessels survival in the rat aorta model. In Vitro 2000;36:336–340.

3 Risau W: Mechanisms of angiogenesis. Nature 1997;386:671–674.

4 Folkman J: What is the evidence that tumors are angiogenesis dependent? J Natl Cancer Inst 1990;82:4–6.

5 Vacca A, Di Loreto M, Ribatti D, Di Stefano R, Gadaleta-Caldarola G, Iodice G, Caloro D, Dammacco F: Bone marrow of patients with active multiple myeloma: Angiogenesis and plasma cell adhesion molecules LFA-1, VLA-4, LAM-1 and CD44. Am J Hematol 1995;50:9–14.

6 Vacca A, Ribatti D, Roncali L, Ranieri G, Serio G, Silvestris F, Dammacco F: Bone marrow angiogenesis and progression in multiple myeloma. Br J Haematol 1994;87:503–508.

7 Geerling S: Kaposi's sarcoma associated with multiple myeloma. South Med J 1994;77:931–932.

8 Warner TF, Krueger RG: Perineural angiogenesis in mice bearing subcutaneous tumours. Br J Exp Pathol 1978;59:282–284.

9 Vacca A, Ribatti D, Presta M, Minischetti M, Iurlaro M, Ria R, Albini A, Bussolino F, Dammacco F: Bone marrow neovascularization, plasma cell angiogenic potential and matrix metalloproteinase-2 secretion parallel progression of human multiple myeloma. Blood 1999; 93:3064–3073.

10 Ohtani H: Stromal reaction in cancer tissue: Pathophysiologic significance of the expression of matrix-degrading enzymes in relation to matrix turnover and immune/inflammatory reaction. Pathol Int 1998;48:1–9.

11 Ribatti D, Gualandris A, Bastaki M, Vacca A, Iurlaro M, Roncali L, Presta M: New model for the study of angiogenesis and antiangiogenesis in the chick embryo chorioallantoic membrane: The gelatin sponge/chorioallantoic membrane assay. J Vasc Res 1997;34:455–463.

12 Menzel T, Rahman Z, Calleja E, White K, Wilson EL, Wieder R, Gabrilove J: Elevated intracellular level of basic fibroblast growth factor correlates with stage of chronic lymphocytic leukemia and is associated with resistance to fludarabine. Blood 1996;87:1056–1063.

13 Børset M, Lien E, Espevik T, Helseth E, Waage A, Sundan A: Concomitant expression of hepatocyte growth factor/scatter factor and the receptor c-MET in human myeloma cell lines. J Biol Chem 1996;271:24655–24661.

14 Børset M, Hjorth-Hansen H, Seidel C, Sundan A, Waage A: Hepatocyte growth factor and its receptor c-met in multiple myeloma. Blood 1996;88:3998–4004.

15 Seidel C, Børset M, Turesson I, Abildgaard N, Sundan A, Waage A: Elevated serum concentrations of hepatocyte growth factor in patients with multiple myeloma. The Nordic Myeloma Study Group. Blood 1998;91:806–812.

16 Bellamy WT, Richter L, Frutiger Y, Grogan TM: Expression of vascular endothelial growth factor and its receptors in hematopoietic malignancies. Blood 1999;59:728–733.

17 Portier M, Zhang XG, Ursule E, Lees D, Jourdan M, Bataille R, Kleine B: Cytokine gene expression in human multiple myeloma. Br J Haematol 1993;85:514–520.

18 Mantovani A, Bussolino F, Dejana E: Cytokine regulation of endothelial cell function. FASEB J 1992;6:2591–2599.

19 Klein B: Cytokine, cytokine receptors, transduction signals and oncogenes in multiple myeloma. Semin Hematol 1995;32:4–19.

20 Merico F, Bergui L, Gregoretti MG, Ghia P, Aimo G, Lindley IJD, Calligaris-Cappio F: Cytokines involved in the progression of multiple myeloma. Clin Exp Immunol 1993;92:27–31.

21 Vacca A, Ribatti D, Iurlaro M, Albini A, Minischetti M, Bussolino F, Pellegrino A, Ria R, Rusnati M, Presta M, Vincenti V, Persico MG, Dammacco F: Human lymphoblastoid cells produce extracellular matrix-degrading enzymes and induce endothelial cell proliferation, migration, morphogenesis and angiogenesis. Int J Clin Lab Res 1998;28:55–68.

22 Huhtala P, Tuuttila A, Chow LT, Lohi J, Keski-Oja J, Tryggvason K: Complete structure of the human gene for 92-kDa type IV collagenase. Divergent regulation of expression for the 92- and 72-kDa enzyme genes in HT-1080 cells. J Biol Chem 1991;266:16485–16490.

23 Vacca A, Ribatti D, Ria R, Pellegrino A, Bruno M, Merchionne F, Dammacco F: Proteolytic activity of human lymphoid tumor cells. Correlation with tumor progression. Dev Immunol 2000;7:77–88.

24 Ribatti D, Vacca A, Nico B, Quondamatteo F, Ria R, Minischetti M, Marzullo A, Herken R, Roncali L, Dammacco F: Bone marrow angiogenesis and mast cell density increase simultaneously with progression of human multiple myeloma. Br J Cancer 1999;79:451–455.

25 Yaccoby S, Barlogie B, Epstein J: Primary myeloma cells growing in SCID-hu mice: A model for studying the biology and the treatment of myeloma and its manifestations. Blood 1998; 92:2908–2913.

26 Vacca A, Ribatti D, Ruco L, Giacchetta F, Nico B, Quondamatteo F, Ria R, Iurlaro M, Dammacco F: Angiogenesis extent and macrophage density increase simultaneously with pathological progression in B-cell non-Hodgkin's lymphomas. Br J Cancer 1999;79:965–970.

27 Leek RD, Lewis CE, Harris AL: The role of macrophages in tumour angiogenesis; in Bicknell R, Lewis CE, Ferrara N (eds): Tumour Angiogenesis. Oxford, Oxford University Press, 1997, pp 81–89.

28 Weidner N: Tumoral vascularity as a prognostic factor in cancer patients: The evidence continues to grow. J Pathol 1998;184:119–122.

29 Hallek M, Bergsagel PL, Anderson KC: Multiple myeloma. Increasing evidence for a multistep transformation process. Blood 1998;91:3–21.

30 Durie BGM: Staging and kinetics of multiple myeloma; in Wiernik PH, Canellos GP, Kyle RA, Schiffer CA (eds): Neoplastic Diseases of the Blood, ed 2. New York, Churchill Livingstone, 1991, vol 1, pp 439–451.

Acta Haematologica

Acta Haematol 2001;106:170–176

Angiogenesis in Acute Myeloid Leukemia and Myelodysplastic Syndrome

Maher Albitar

Department of Leukemia and Hematopathology, University of Texas, M.D. Anderson Cancer Center, Houston, Tex., USA

Key Words
Angiogenesis · Fibroblast growth factor, basic · Hepatocyte growth factor · Leukemia · Neovascularization · Receptors · Tumor necrosis factor-α · Vascular endothelial growth factor

Abstract
Increased angiogenesis is important in the pathophysiology of solid tumors. Recent studies show that angiogenesis and angiogenic factors play an important role in hematological malignancies. Both acute myeloid leukemia (AML) and myelodysplastic syndrome (MDS) are associated with a substantial increase in vascularity in the bone marrow as well as increased levels of various angiogenic factors including vascular endothelial growth factor (VEGF), basic fibroblast growth factor, angiogenin, angiopoietin-1, platelet-derived growth factor, hepatocyte growth factor, epidermal growth factor, tumor necrosis factor-α, and transforming growth factor-α and transforming growth factor-β. Most of these angiogenic factors appear to be secreted by the neoplastic hematopoietic cells and appear to promote the growth and proliferation of the leukemic cells in an autocrine fashion. More importantly, angiogenic factors play a role in the clinical behavior and outcome of both AML and MDS. Despite significant overlap between MDS and AML in many aspects, higher levels of cellular VEGF and lower levels KDR are seen in MDS than in AML. Antiangiogenic therapy may play a role in AML and MDS and some differences in response may exist between MDS and AML.

Introduction

Neovascularization is an important factor in the growth and proliferation of solid tumors [1–5], but its importance in hematological neoplasms has been realized only recently [6–9]. Hematological malignancies are unique because a significant overlap between endothelial and hematopoietic systems has been established; numerous publications have reported on the role of angiogenic factors in the growth and differentiation of hematopoietic cells [10–12]. This raises the possibility that overexpression of angiogenic factors in leukemias serves two purposes: first, promoting growth and proliferation of the hematopoietic cells through direct effects, and second, providing neovascularization, which in turn helps the growth and proliferation of hematopoietic cells. Since cells in acute myeloid leukemia (AML) and myelodysplastic syndrome (MDS) are generally immersed in blood, it is not clear whether neovascularization is an 'innocent bystander' or a necessary factor for the growth of neoplastic

KARGER

Fax + 41 61 306 12 34
E-Mail karger@karger.ch
www.karger.com

0001–5792/01/1064–0170$17.50/0

Accessible online at:
www.karger.com/journals/aha

Maher Albitar, MD
Department of Hematopathology, University of Texas, M.D. Anderson Cancer Center
1515 Holcombe Boulevard, Box 72
Houston, TX 77030-4095 (USA)
Tel. +1 713 794 1292, Fax +1 713 794 1800, E-Mail malbitar@mdanderson.org

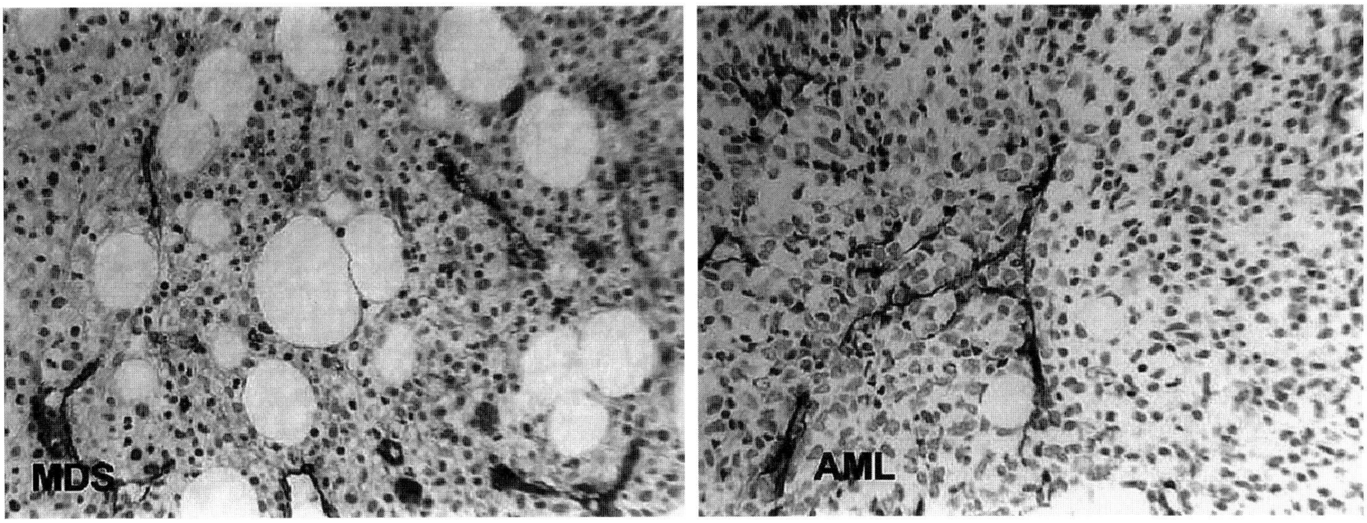

Fig. 1. Increased vascularity in AML and MDS. Representative immunohistochemical staining for anti-factor VIII in bone marrow sections from patients with AML and MDS.

Table 1. Increased neovascularization in AML and MDS

	Blood vessels (MVD)		Relative vessel area		Correlation with BM cellularity (p value)
	number	p value	median %	p value	
Control	11.2		2.8		
AML	16.1	0.02	4.3	0.23	0.33
MDS	20.4	0.0004	5.2	0.06	0.74

MVD = Microvessel density.

cells in these two diseases. A further complication is that most angiogenic factors are response factors to the inflammatory process [13], which may also arise as a result of leukemogenesis, and it is possible that neovascularization in AML and MDS is simply an inflammatory response rather than an active and necessary process for the neoplasia.

In this article, I will attempt to describe the changes in angiogenic factors and neovascularization in AML and MDS. Although I believe that AML and MDS are two separate diseases, they overlap considerably, both clinically and biologically. Whenever possible, I will describe the differences in angiogenic changes between AML and MDS and demonstrate that angiogenesis and angiogenic factors play an active role in the biology and clinical behavior of these two diseases, regardless of whether angiogenesis is a response to the leukemic process or an essential process necessary for leukemogenesis.

Increased Vascularity in AML and MDS

Padro et al. [8], Hussong et al. [9], and our group [6] have reported increased vascularity in AML; we also reported this finding in MDS. As shown in table 1 and figure 1, vascularity increases substantially in the bone marrow (BM) of patients with AML and MDS. The level of this vascularity does not appear to correlate with the cellularity of the BM, which suggests that vascularity is not a direct result of the increased BM cellularity in AML and MDS. We measured not only the number of blood vessels in BM but also the relative vascular spaces on the BM biopsies. The number of blood vessels increased substantially, but the vascular spaces did not. Possibly this is due to the collapse of blood vessels induced by the increased cellularity. This hypothesis is supported by the finding that after initiating therapy (day 14 on therapy), the number of blood vessels does not change, but the vascular spaces increase significantly (fig. 2a, b). This dilatation in the blood vessels disappears when BM is examined at later stages (> day 15 after initiation of therapy). We saw no significant difference in neovascularization between AML and MDS.

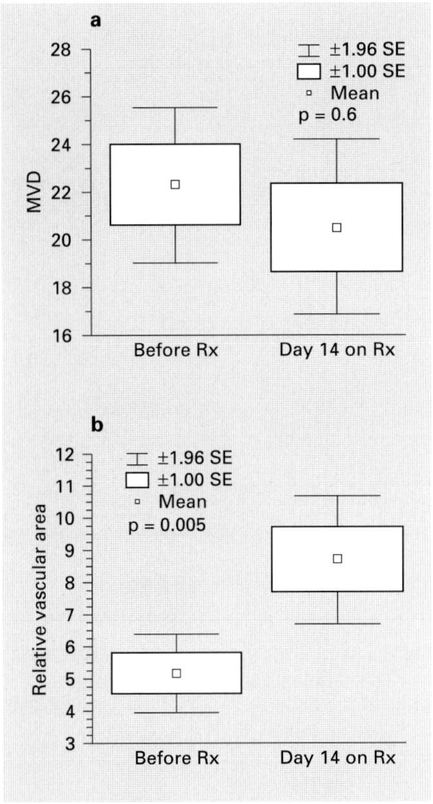

Fig. 2. Changes in vascularity with therapy. The box plots compare the number of blood vessels (MVD = microvessel density) (**a**) and relative vascular area (**b**) before therapy with those on day 14 on therapy (Rx).

Angiogenic Factors in Plasma of Patients with AML and MDS

Numerous growth factors have been reported to be angiogenic factors that promote the growth of endothelial cells [13–20], most of them also promote the growth of hematopoietic cells [21, 22]. These factors include vascular endothelial growth factor (VEGF), basic fibroblast growth factor (bFGF), angiogenin, angiopoietin-1, platelet-derived growth factor, hepatocyte growth factor (HGF), epidermal growth factor, insulin-like growth factor-1, tumor necrosis factor-α (TNF-α), transforming growth factors-α and -β (TGF-α, TGF-β), interleukin 6 (IL-6), interleukin 8 (IL-8), and granulocyte-macrophage colony-stimulating factor [13].

Most of these factors have been reported to be increased in the sera of patients with AML and MDS [23–25], although variations in the levels of various angiogenic factors and in their clinical importance have been reported. This variation between reports is due to a difference between serum and plasma levels. Some of these factors are expressed at relatively high levels in circulating leukemic cells and platelets [26, 27]. Because these factors can be squeezed out of the platelets and cells in the process of serum formation and clotting of blood samples, serum levels may depend on the number of platelets and circulating cells. This is a more serious issue in patients with leukemia and MDS than it is in patients with solid tumors because of the variation between patients in the number of circulating cells and platelets in AML and MDS.

Several investigators [28, 29] as well as our group [6] demonstrated that plasma is a more reliable source for analyzing angiogenic factor in patients with leukemia. Table 2 illustrates the levels of some of the angiogenic factors in patients with AML and MDS seen in our institution. All of these values are derived from plasma and do

Table 2. Levels of angiogenic factors in AML and MDS

Angiogenic factor	Control pg/ml	AML pg/ml	MDS pg/ml
VEGF	26.74 (23.17–53.88)	30.43 (21.47–439.25)	31.05 (22.45–408.7)
FGF	5.37 (4.56–13.65)	6.48 (4.66–203.74)	6.61 (4.7–49.74)
HGF	336.1 (164–522)	899.6 (101.9–12,819)	737.6 (192.3–3,533.6)
TNF-α	8.6 (7.1–10.3)	8.9 (7.3–19)	8.4 (7.1–11.7)
TGF-α	0	0 (0–199.4)	0
Angiogenin	197,072 (123,900–314,720)	587,200 (127,620–1,054,000)	632,170 (280,200–926,600)

Figures represent median with the range in parentheses.

3

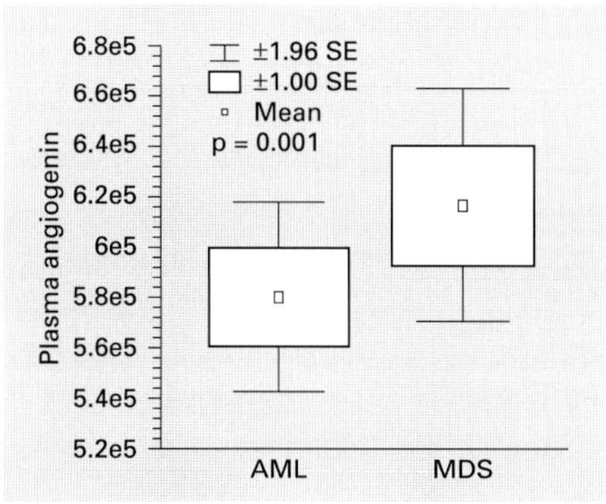

4

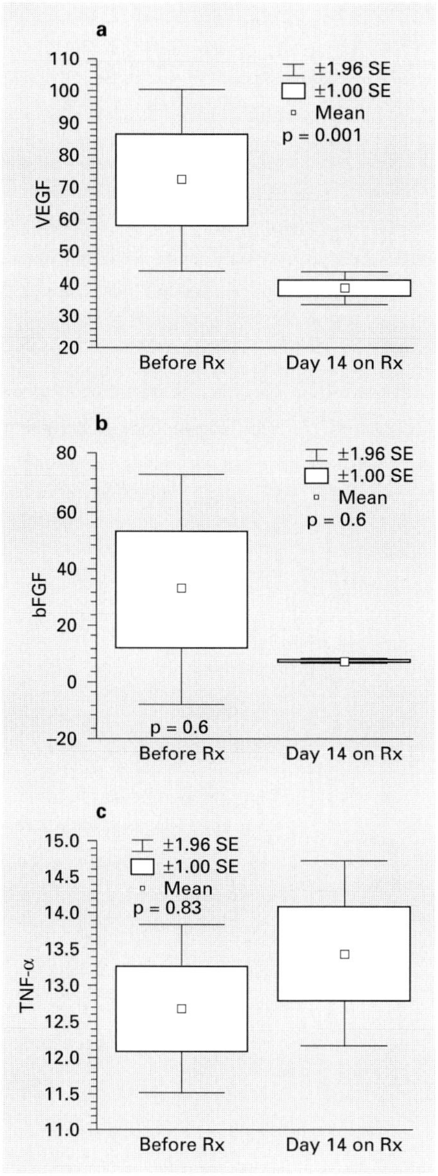

5

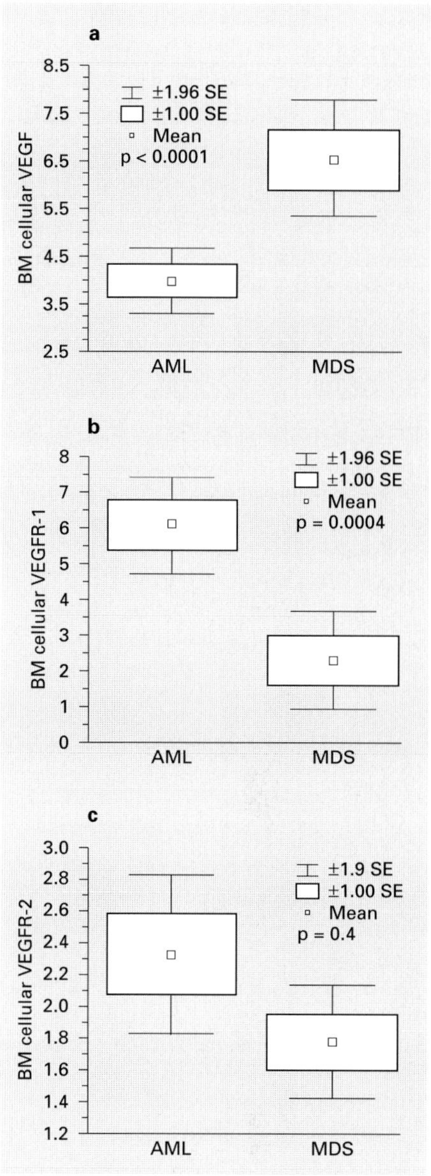

Fig. 3. Higher levels of angiogenin in MDS. This box plot shows that significantly higher levels of angiogenin are found in MDS than in AML ($p = 0.001$, Kruskal-Wallis test).
Fig. 4. Changes in angiogenic factors with therapy. Levels of VEGF (**a**) and bFGF (**b**) were reduced after therapy ($p = 0.001$ and $p = 0.06$, respectively). No reduction was seen in the levels of TNF-α ($p = 0.83$) (**c**).
Fig. 5. Differences between AML and MDS in the levels of cellular VEGF and its receptors. Significantly higher levels of VEGF are detected in MDS than in AML (**a**), but lower levels of VEGFR-1 are found in MDS than in AML (**b**); no significant difference was detected between AML and MDS in the levels of VEGFR-2 (**c**).

not appear to be affected greatly by freezing and thawing. However, some variation was observed in the same patients when several samples were obtained at different times. Most studies, including ours, report total rather than free levels of angiogenic factors. This is particularly important because free circulating receptors that may bind to these angiogenic factors are often present and the net effect may depend on levels of free angiogenic factors rather than on the total level [30, 31]. For example, circulating Flt-1 protein, which is a receptor for the VEGF, has been detected, and it may bind to circulating VEGF, suppressing its effects [30, 31].

When we compared the levels of various plasma angiogenic factors in AML with those in MDS, we found no significant differences in the levels of VEGF, bFGF, TNF-α, TGF-β, HGF, IL-6, epidermal growth factor, IL-8, or endostatin. Angiogenin levels were significantly higher in MDS than they were in AML (fig. 3).

We also investigated the changes in the levels of some angiogenic factors in patients with AML and MDS during therapy. When we compared levels before therapy with those afterward, we found that VEGF and bFGF levels were significantly reduced at around day 14 of therapy (fig. 4a, b). In contrast, TNF-α levels did not change sig-

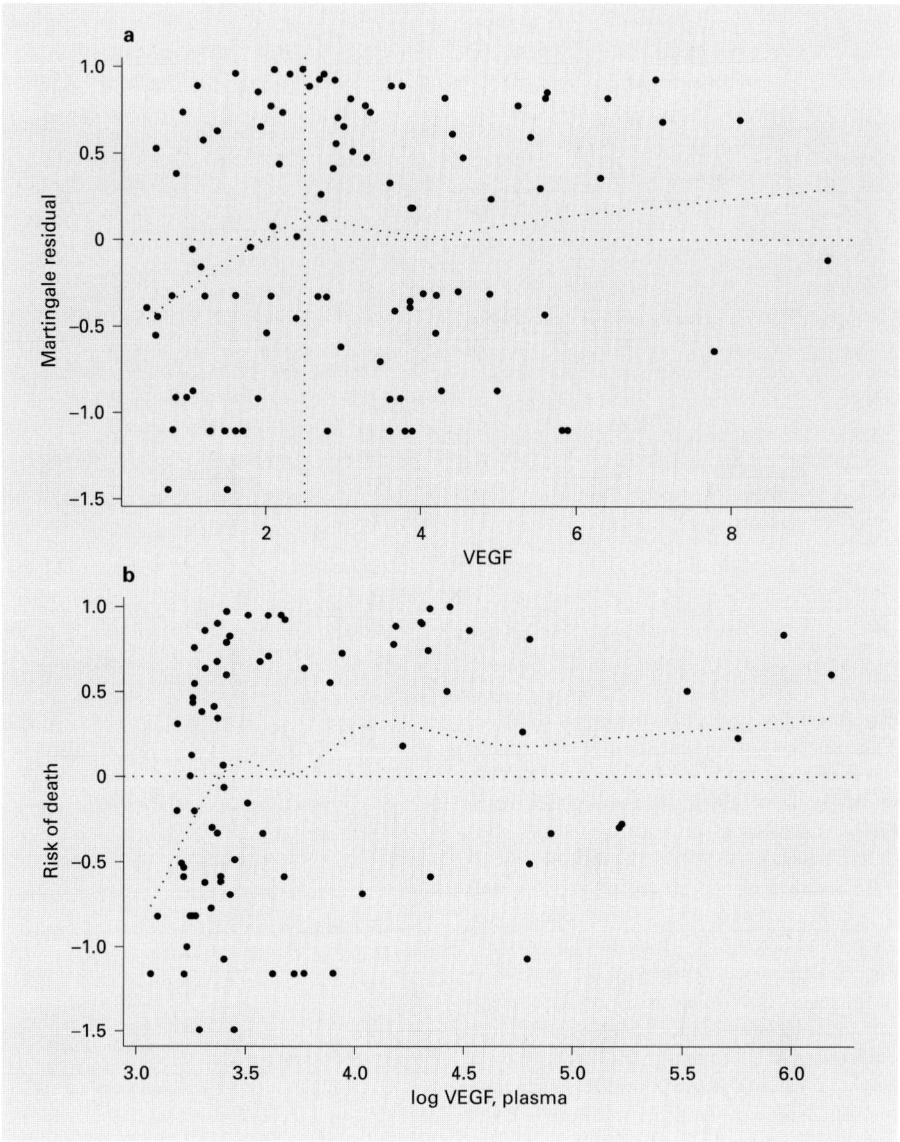

Fig. 6. Correlation between VEGF levels and survival in AML. Martingale residual plots correlating cellular (**a**) and plasma (**b**) levels of VEGF with relative risk of death. The risk of death (above 0) increases with increasing levels of VEGF.

nificantly (fig. 4c). These findings support the hypothesis that leukemic cells are most likely the source of most of the plasma angiogenic factors.

Expression of Angiogenic Factors in Leukemic Cells

Several investigators, including our group, have reported the detection of VEGF and its receptors 1 and 2 (VEGFR-1, or Flt-1, and VEGFR-2, or KDR, respectively) in leukemic cells from patients with AML and MDS [32–35]. This suggests that angiogenic factors secreted by the leukemic cells themselves may promote their own growth and proliferation in paracrine fashion. We have reported that high levels of VEGF, VEGFR-1, and VEGFR-2 can be detected in leukemic cells in BM from patients with AML and MDS with some variation between patients. It is interesting that significantly higher levels of VEGF protein were detected in MDS BM cells than in AML BM cells ($p < 0.0001$, Kruskal-Wallis test) (fig. 5a), whereas in contrast with those results, we found significantly lower levels of VEGFR-1 (Flt-1) in MDS than in AML BM cells ($p = 0.0004$, Kruskal-Wallis test) (fig. 5b) and no significantly different levels of VEGFR-2 (KDR) between AML and MDS ($p = 0.4$, Kruskal-Wallis test) (fig. 5c). These differences could be because the dominant cell populations in AML are blasts whereas those in MDS are maturing cells. Nevertheless, we have demonstrated that VEGF and its receptors are expressed in significantly higher levels in MDS than in normal BM, despite the relative similarity in cell population and maturation.

Clinical Relevance of Angiogenesis in AML and MDS

Although no evidence to date has suggested that the level of neovascularization in BM correlates with specific clinical behavior or response to therapy in AML or MDS, this may change as new therapeutic approaches against angiogenesis are used in these diseases. A correlation between various angiogenic factors and clinical behavior has been reported in several studies [6, 7, 35]. We have reported that higher levels of cellular VEGF in the BM cells from patients with AML correlate with more aggressive disease [35]. To determine the prognostic significance of cellular VEGF, we examined the martingale residual plots (fig. 6a, b). Residual values above 0 correspond to a relative risk of death above 1; those below 0 correspond to a relative risk of death of less than 1. Survival probability reduced continuously as intracellular VEGF increased up to about 2.5, after which there was no further effect on survival (fig. 6b). We obtained similar results when we used plasma levels of VEGF (fig. 6b). Furthermore, high plasma levels of HGF, bFGF, IL-6, and endostatin all correlated with shorter survival in AML with current standard therapy for this disease [36].

The presence of a correlation between angiogenic factors and clinical behavior suggests that these factors play an important role in the biology of AML and MDS. The challenge at this point is to develop new therapeutic approaches that specifically inactivate the angiogenic factors and suppress the growth and proliferation of leukemic cells.

In summary, angiogenic factors and neovascularization are increased in AML and MDS. The overlap between angiogenesis and hematopoiesis makes targeting angiogenesis in the therapy of AML and MDS an intriguing approach. More research is needed to understand and dissect the complex interaction between various angiogenic factors and possible variation between individual patients.

References

1 Fanelli M, Locopo N, Gattuso D, Gasparini G: Assessment of tumor vascularization: Immunohistochemical and non-invasive methods. Int J Biol Markers 1999;14:218–231.
2 Samejima N, Yamazaki K: A study on the vascular proliferation in tissues around the tumor in breast cancer. Jpn J Surg 1988;18:235–242.
3 Edel MJ, Robbins PD, Papadimitriou JM, D'Antuono MF, Harvey JM, Mitchel CA, Dawkins HJ: Assessment of vascularity in breast carcinoma by computer-assisted video analysis (CAVA) and its association with axillary lymph node status. Breast Cancer Res Treat 1998;47:17–27.
4 Piérard GE, Piérard-Franchimont C: Stochastic relationship between the growth fraction and vascularity of thin malignant melanomas. Eur J Cancer 1997;33:1888–1892.
5 Tanigawa N, Matsumura M, Amaya H, Kitaoka A, Shimomatsuya T, Lu C, Muraoka R, Tanaka T: Tumor vascularity correlates with the prognosis of patients with esophageal squamous cell carcinoma. Cancer 1997;79:220–225.
6 Aguayo A, Kantarjian H, Manshouri T, Gidel C, Estey E, Thomas D, Koller C, Estrov Z, O'Brien S, Keating M, Freireich E, Albitar M: Angiogenesis in acute and chronic leukemias and myelodysplastic syndromes. Blood 2000; 96:2240–2245.
7 Perez-Atayde AR, Sallan SE, Tedrow U, Connors S, Allred E, Folkman J: Spectrum of tumor angiogenesis in the bone marrow of children with acute lymphoblastic leukemia. Am J Pathol 1997;50:815–821.
8 Padro T, Ruiz S, Bieker R, Burger H, Steins M, Kienast J, Buchner T, Berdel WE, Mesters RM: Increased angiogenesis in the bone marrow of patients with acute myeloid leukemia. Blood 2000;95:2637–2644.
9 Hussong JW, Rodgers GM, Shami PJ: Evidence of increased angiogenesis in patients with acute myeloid leukemia. Blood 2000;95: 309–313.
10 Orkin SH, Porcher C, Fujiwara Y, Visvader J, Wang LC: Intersections between blood cell development and leukemia genes. Cancer Res 1999;59(7 suppl):1784–1788.
11 Crosby JR, Kaminski WE, Schatteman G, Martin PJ, Raines EW, Seifert RA, Bowen-Pope DF: Endothelial cells of hematopoietic origin make a significant contribution to adult blood vessel formation. Circ Res 2000;87:728–730.
12 Ribatti D, Vacca A, Roncali L, Dammacco F: Hematopoiesis and angiogenesis: A link between two apparently independent processes. J Hematother Stem Cell Res 2000;9:13–19.
13 Mangi MH, Newland AC: Angiogenesis and angiogenic mediators in haematological malignancies. Br J Haematol 2000;111:43–51.
14 Bellamy WT, Richter L, Frutiger Y, Grogan TM: Expression of vascular endothelial growth factor and its receptors in hematopoietic malignancies. Cancer Res 1999;59:728–733.
15 Allouche M: Basic fibroblast growth factor and hematopoiesis. Leukemia 1995;96:937–942.
16 Allouche M, Bikfalvi A: The role of fibroblast growth factor-2 (FGF-2) in hematopoiesis. Prog Growth Factor Res 1995;6:35–48.
17 Bikfalvi A, Han ZC: Angiogenic factors are hematopoietic growth factors and vice versa. Leukemia 1994;8:523–529.
18 Gerwins P, Skoldenberg E, Claesson-Welsh L: Function of fibroblast growth factors and vascular endothelial growth factors and their receptors in angiogenesis. Crit Rev Oncol Hematol 2000;34:185–194.
19 Sensebe L, Deschaseaux M, Li J, Hervé P, Charbord P: The broad spectrum of cytokine gene expression by myoid cells from the human marrow microenvironment. Stem Cells 1997; 15:133–143.
20 Schott RJ, Morrow LA: Growth factors and angiogenesis. Cardiovasc Res 1993;27:1155–1161.

21 Visvader JE, Fujiwara Y, Orkin SH: Unsuspected role for the T-cell leukemia protein SCL/tal-1 in vascular development. Genes Dev 1998;12:47347–47349.

22 Pruneri G, Bertolini F, Soligo D, Carboni N, Cortelezzi A, Ferrucci PF, Buffa R, Lambertenghi-Deliliers G, Pezzella F: Angiogenesis in myelodysplastic syndromes. Br J Cancer 1999; 81:1398–1401.

23 Kitagawa M, Saito I, Kuwata T, Yoshida S, Yamaguchi S, Takahashi M, Tanizawa T, Kamiyama R, Hirokawa K: Overexpression of tumor necrosis factor (TNF)-alpha and interferon (IFN)-gamma by bone marrow cells from patients with myelodysplastic syndromes. Leukemia 1997;11:2049–2054.

24 Tobler A, Moser B, Dewald B, Geiser T, Studer H, Baggiolini M, Fey MF: Constitutive expression of interleukin-8 and its receptor in human myeloid and lymphoid leukemia. Blood 1993; 82:2517–2525.

25 Salven P, Orpana A, Joensuu H: Leukocytes and platelets of patients with cancer contain high levels of vascular endothelial growth factor. Clin Cancer Res 1999;5:487–491.

26 Martyre MC, Le Bousse-Kerdiles MC, Romquin N, Chevillard S, Praloran V, Demory JL, Dupriez B: Elevated levels of basic fibroblast growth factor in megakaryocytes and platelets from patients with idiopathic myelofibrosis. Br J Haematol 1997;97:441–448.

27 Lee JK, Hong YJ, Han CJ, Hwang DY, Hong SI: Clinical usefulness of serum and plasma vascular endothelial growth factor in cancer patients: Which is the optimal specimen? Int J Oncol 2000;17:149–152.

28 Gunsilius E, Gastl G: Platelets and VEGF blood levels in cancer patients. Br J Cancer 1999;81:185–186.

29 Hornig C, Barleon B, Ahmad S, Vuorela P, Ahmed A, Weich HA: Release and complex formation of soluble VEGFR-1 from endothelial cells and biological fluids. Lab Invest 2000; 80:443–454.

30 Vuorela P, Helske S, Hornig C, Alitalo K, Weich H, Halmesmaki E: Amniotic fluid-soluble vascular endothelial growth factor receptor-1 in preeclampsia. Obstet Gynecol 2000;95: 353-357.

31 Ziegler BL, Valtieri M, Porada GA, De Maria R, Muller R, Masella B, Gabbianelli M, Casella I, Pelosi E, Bock T, Zanjani ED, Peschle C: KDR receptor: A key marker defining hematopoietic stem cells. Science 1999;285:1553–1558.

32 Peichev M, Naiyer AJ, Pereira D, Zhu Z, Lane WJ, Williams M, Oz MC, Hicklin DJ, Witte L, Moore MA, Rafii S: Expression of VEGFR-2 and AC133 by circulating human CD34(+) cells identifies a population of functional endothelial precursors. Blood 2000;95:952–958.

33 Dias S, Hattori K, Zhu Z, Heissig B, Choy M, Lane W, Wu Y, Chadburn A, Hyjek E, Gill M, Hicklin DJ, Witte L, Moore MA, Rafii S: Autocrine stimulation of VEGFR-2 activates human leukemic cell growth and migration. J Clin Invest 2000;106:511–521.

34 Borset M, Seidel C, Hjorth-Hansen H, Waage A, Sundan A: The role of hepatocyte growth factor and its receptor c-Met in multiple myeloma and other blood malignancies. Leuk Lymphoma 1999;32:249–256.

35 Aguayo A, Kantarjian H, Manshouri T, Gidel C, Keating M, Giles F, Estrov Z, Barlogie B, Estey E, Albitar M: Cellular VEGF is an independent predictor of outcome in patients with acute myeloid leukemia. Blood 1999;94:3717–3721.

36 Albitar M, Estey E, Cortes J, O'Brien S, Giles F, Kurzrock R: Prognostic significance of cytokine levels in newly-diagnosed AML and high-risk myelodysplasia. Submitted.

Acta Hæmatologica

Acta Haematol 2001;106:177–183

Angiogenesis in Chronic Myeloproliferative Diseases

Francesco Di Raimondo[a] Giuseppe A. Palumbo[a] Stefano Molica[b] Rosario Giustolisi[a]

[a]Institute of Hematology, University of Catania, and [b]Division of Clinical Hematology and Oncology, Azienda Ospedaliera 'Pugliese-Ciaccio', Catanzaro, Italy

Key Words

Angiogenesis · Myelofibrosis · Chronic myeloid leukemia · Essential thrombocythemia · Polycythemia vera

Abstract

Increased angiogenic activity has been demonstrated in myelofibrosis with myeloid metaplasia (MMM), chronic myeloid leukemia (CML), and essential thrombocythemia (ET) by both bone marrow microvessel density evaluation and measurement of circulating angiogenic factors. MMM is probably the disease with the more pronounced angiogenesis among myeloproliferative disorders but the significance of this finding remains speculative since the angiogenic activity is not correlated with any of the clinical and laboratory features of the disease. Circulating serum levels of angiogenic factors such as vascular endothelial growth factor (VEGF) and hepatocyte growth factor (HGF) were found increased in MMM, CML and ET but the frequent thrombocytosis that accompanies these diseases could limit the interpretation of these data since platelets and megakaryocytes may be considered a major source at least for VEGF. However, CML patients treated with interferon were found to have lower VEGF and HGF levels than untreated or hydroxyurea-treated patients, thus suggesting a possible antiangiogenic mechanism of this drug. In addition, preliminary experiences with the antiangiogenic drug thalidomide have shown therapeutic activity in some myeloproliferative disorders.

Introduction

The field of neoangiogenesis has for a long time been an active area of research relating to solid tumors [1] but the interest of the hematological scientific community in studying the angiogenesis phenomena has started only in 1997, when Folkman's group demonstrated that bone marrow (BM) of children affected by acute lymphoblastic leukemia contained many more microvessels than normal BM [2]. Before that time scanty observations were reported in the literature demonstrating an increase of vascularity in the BM of other hematological diseases. Examples of these observations are the paper published by Vacca et al. [3] (1994), dealing with angiogenesis in multiple myeloma, and the even older publication by Thiele et al. [4] (1992) that showed an increase of vascular architecture in BM of patients affected by myelofibrosis and polycythemia vera (PV). Therefore, by looking over the literature, the increased vascular density in the BM of myeloproliferative disorders is not a new finding. However, this observation remained isolated until the hematologists started to be interested in a systematic study of angiogene-

KARGER

Fax + 41 61 306 12 34
E-Mail karger@karger.ch
www.karger.com

0001–5792/01/1064–0177$17.50/0

Accessible online at:
www.karger.com/journals/aha

Dr. F. Di Raimondo
Institute of Hematology, Ospedale Ferrarotto
V. Citelli 6, I–95124 Catania (Italy)
Tel. +39 095 743 59 69, Fax +39 095 731 15 10
E-Mail diraimon@sirio-oncology.it

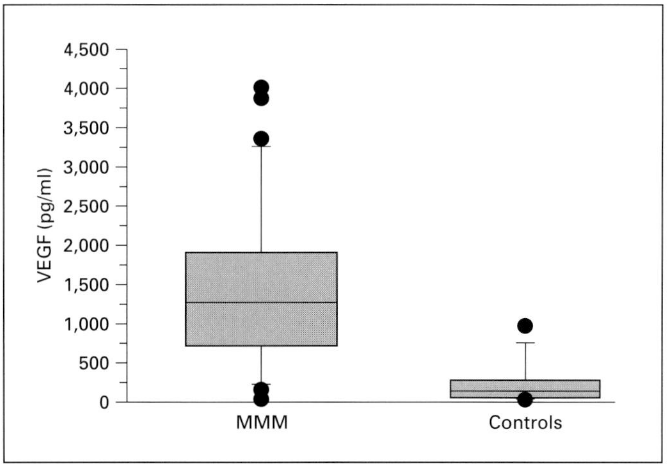

Fig. 1. Serum VEGF levels in MMM patients and normal controls. 10th, 25th, 50th, 75th and 90th percentiles are indicated by horizontal lines. Boxed areas indicate values between 25th and 75th percentiles [15].

sis and a confirmation of this finding was published only in July 2000, when Lundberg et al. [5] showed that BM of PV, chronic myelocytic leukemia (CML) and myelofibrosis with myeloid metaplasia (MMM) has an increased vascularity. This study also showed that the vessels of myeloproliferative diseases are more tortuous and branched than normal controls. In addition, the percentage of cells that stained for vascular endothelial growth factor (VEGF) was increased in respect to controls and there was a significant correlation between VEGF-positive cells and the number of microvessels.

Myelofibrosis

The study of Lundberg et al. [5] has shown that the increased vascular density, the positivity for VEGF staining and the tortuosity of the vessels were more pronounced in MMM than in the other myeloproliferative disorders. Therefore, MMM seems to be the paradigmatic disease for studying angiogenesis in myeloproliferative diseases. In fact a recent study on 114 patients affected by MMM conducted at the Mayo Clinic and reported by Mesa et al. [6] has shown that 70% of MMM patients had a substantial increase of BM microvessel density (MVD). The increase of MVD was much more pronounced not only in respect to normal controls but also when compared with patients affected by PV or essential thrombocythemia (ET). This study has also shown that the increased angiogenesis has a prognostic significance. Survival was significantly shorter in patients with more marked BM MVD and univariate and multivariate analyses have identified BM angiogenesis as the stronger parameter, together with age, affecting survival. The current knowledge in MMM biology indicates that the clinical features of this disease are derived not only from a clonal myeloid proliferation but also from an abnormal cytokine release that induces a BM stromal reaction with subsequent fibrosis [7]. Therefore, many cytokines are implicated in the MMM pathogenesis and several studies have reported that patients affected by MMM have increased circulating levels of transforming growth factor-β, basic fibroblast growth factor (bFGF), and platelet-derived growth factor that, beside other activities, are strong inducers of angiogenesis [8–11]. Measurements of these or other more vascular-specific cytokines may be a valid alternative to the measurement of angiogenesis by MVD count that, although it is an accepted way of evaluating angiogenesis [12], has the limitation of a lack of objectivity and is not suitable for frequent measurements. Many circulating angiogenic factors have been identified but so far the role and contribution of each of them in tumoral angiogenesis is not clear. VEGF seems to be one of the most important mediators of both normal and tumoral angiogenesis [13]; indeed, the good preclinical results obtained by blocking VEGF or its receptors indicate that this factor may have a leading position in the hierarchy of angiogenesis mediators [14]. On this basis we evaluated the serum levels of VEGF in 31 patients affected by MMM and in 12 healthy subjects and correlated VEGF concentration with clinical and laboratory features of disease [15].

We found that MMM patients had much higher concentrations of circulating VEGF than controls (median 1,208 vs. 138 ng/ml, $p < 0.0001$) (fig. 1). No correlation was found between VEGF and Hb, WBC, Plt, LDH, creatinine, BM cellularity, fibrosis, splenomegaly, hepatomegaly and therapy. However, in the subgroup of patients with a normal or low VEGF concentration, a direct correlation between VEGF and platelet count ($r = 0.90$, $p = 0.002$) was detected. Moreover, patients with a platelet count $<300 \times 10^9$/l had VEGF serum levels lower than patients with a higher Plt count (median VEGF 864 vs. 1,557 pg/ml, $p = 0.001$). In 6 patients and in 8 controls we also measured VEGF in the plasma and we observed that the VEGF concentration was much higher in platelet-rich than in platelet-poor plasma and that platelets of MMM patients contained and/or released 4 times more VEGF than those of healthy controls. These results indicate that

VEGF is overproduced in MMM and that platelets are probably a major source of VEGF. This is an expected finding since it has been demonstrated that normal megakaryocytes contain both VEGF mRNA and protein; in addition to the synthesized VEGF they endocytose and concentrate circulating VEGF, which is later transported to alpha granules [16], and it is well known that there is a large number of megakaryocytes in MMM BM. However, since in MMM both platelets and megakaryocytes may be larger than normal, it is possible that MMM platelets contain more VEGF just because of their bigger size. In any case, these findings highlight the central role for megakaryocytes as a source for cytokine-mediated BM stromal reaction in MMM. However, other cells, also involved in clot formation, must be involved in the production of the very high level of VEGF found in MMM patients. In our study, in fact, the VEGF serum levels were always higher than the platelet-rich plasma levels and the 4-fold difference in platelet-contained VEGF cannot explain by itself the 10-fold difference in circulating VEGF concentrations between MMM patients and healthy controls.

Although these data clearly demonstrated an increased angiogenesis in MMM, the role of this finding in the pathogenesis of the disease is not clear. In the study of Mesa et al. [6] the increased BM vascularity was associated with marked splenomegaly and the authors speculated that the increased angiogenesis may facilitate extramedullary hematopoiesis by favoring the migration of BM hematological precursors into the systemic circulation and subsequent seeding in the spleen. The increase of serum VEGF found in our study could be in line with this hypothesis because this factor has been characterized for its ability to promote vascular leak and permeability and was in fact originally termed vascular permeability factor [13]. In addition, recent studies indicate that pluripotent hemopoietic stem cells express receptors for VEGF [17]. Therefore, it is possible that the massive amount of circulating VEGF in MMM could have an effect on the excessive production and/or migration of the large number of circulating hemopoietic precursors in the peripheral blood that is a typical feature of MMM. In this light, in 18 MMM patients we also evaluated the hepatocyte growth factor (HGF) serum level. HGF has in fact well-known angiogenic properties and is also called scatter factor because of its ability to promote migration of the target cells [18]. We found that MMM have much higher HGF levels than controls and that there was a good correlation between VEGF and HGF levels ($r = 0.69$, $p = 0.001$) thus confirming the involvement of HGF in the process of angiogenesis. However, preliminary data from our laboratory have not shown any correlation between the concentration of VEGF or HGF and the percentage of CD34-positive cells in the peripheral blood of MMM patients, thus suggesting that the feature of increased hematopoietic progenitors in peripheral blood of MMM patients is not dependent on angiogenic factor serum concentrations (unpubl. data).

The demonstration that neoangiogenesis is an important feature of MMM and may have prognostic significance has provided the rationale for clinical investigations with antiangiogenic drugs and preliminary results have shown that thalidomide may have a therapeutic activity in some Philadelphia-negative myeloproliferative disorders, including MMM [19].

Chronic Myeloid Leukemia

After the first report by Lundberg et al. [5] showing an increased MVD in myeloproliferative diseases, including CML, the same group has extended the study of angiogenesis by measuring the intracellular expression of VEGF and bFGF in BM of 13 CML patients and they found that, beside an increase of MVD, these patients had an higher concentration of VEGF, but not bFGF, than normal controls [20]. Relevant data dealing with this subject also came from a study conducted at the M.D. Anderson Cancer Center [21], where several hematological malignancies (chronic lymphocytic leukemia, CML, acute lymphocytic leukemia, acute myeloid leukemia, myelodysplastic syndrome) were tested at diagnosis for the BM vascularity and the plasma concentration of some angiogenic factors. The result of this study was that CML was among the diseases with the largest number of BM vessels and it came first when the relative areas of vascular beds in the BM of various diseases were calculated (it should be pointed out that in this study MMM patients were not included). In addition, this study demonstrated that CML patients had higher plasma levels of VEGF, bFGF, HGF, and TNF-α than normal controls.

Actually, an increase of circulating angiogenic factors is a finding which can be expected, since it has been demonstrated by in vitro experiments that primary-derived CML cells and CML cell lines may secrete VEGF, HGF, bFGF and IL-8 [22, 23]. In this light, we have evaluated the serum concentrations of VEGF and HGF in 30 CML patients in different phases of the disease [24]. We found that in half of these patients the concentration of both factors was higher than the upper normal limit and the

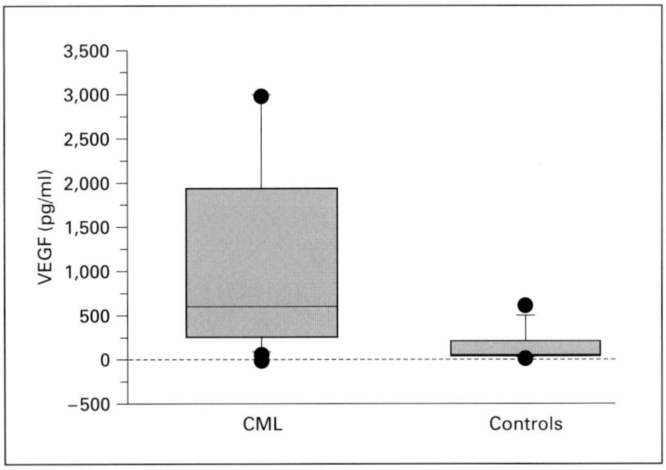

Fig. 2. Serum VEGF levels in CML patients and normal controls. 10th, 25th, 50th, 75th and 90th percentiles are indicated by horizontal lines. Boxed areas indicate values between 25th and 75th percentiles.

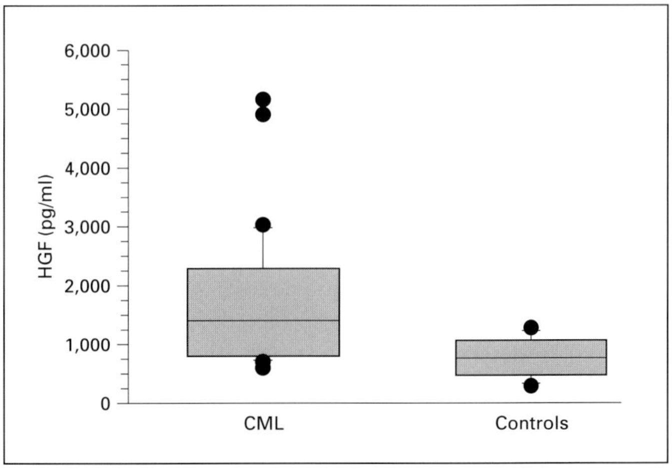

Fig. 3. Serum HGF levels in CML patients and normal controls. 10th, 25th, 50th, 75th and 90th percentiles are indicated by horizontal lines. Boxed areas indicate values between 25th and 75th percentiles.

median values of VEGF and HGF were significantly higher than in normal controls (p = 0.004 and 0.01 for VEGF and HGF, respectively) (fig. 2, 3). VEGF also correlated with Plt count (r = 0.70, p = 0.0001) and WBC count (r = 0.54, p = 0.002) while HGF showed a good correlation with most of the parameters expressing tumor burden such as WBC count (r = 0.83, p = 0.0001), LDH (r = 0.71, p = 0.0001), splenomegaly (r = 0.66, p = 0.0001), hepatomegaly (r = 0.50, p = 0.005), and Hb (r = –0.65, p = 0.0001). There was quite a good correlation (r = 0.48, p = 0.008) between the two factors, while none of the two factors correlated with the erythropoietin serum levels, indicating that the increase of these factors was not secondary to hypoxia that can be present in anemic patients [25]. In addition, we found that levels of both VEGF and HGF were lower in patients at diagnosis or in the early chronic phase compared to patients in the late chronic phase or with accelerated disease but the difference was not statistically significant. In contrast, a significant difference was found when we divided our patients according to treatment: IFN-treated patients had a much lower value of both factors than hydroxyurea-treated and untreated patients (median value of VEGF 293 vs. 1,244, p = 0.01; median value of HGF 816 vs. 2,038, p = 0.005). These data indicate that the serum level of angiogenic factors is increased in CML patients and that the complex antitumor mechanisms of action of IFN in CML may include the inhibition of some important soluble mediators of angiogenesis. Similar results were reported by Willer et al. [26] who found that IFN-treated CML patients had a significant lower BM MVD than patients at diagnosis.

ET and PV

The clinical significance of BM vascularity and plasma levels of angiogenic factors individually or combined has recently also been investigated in ET. Mesa et al. [27] looked at the extent and clinical relevance of BM angiogenesis in 164 ET patients. Quantitative evaluation of angiogenesis was carried out on BM trephine biopsies highlighted by immunohistochemistry using an antibody with CD34 specificity. BM angiogenesis was significantly higher in ET patients in comparison to either normal controls or reactive thrombocytosis. From a clinical point of view an increased BM angiogenesis in ET correlated with splenomegaly and forecasted transformation towards postthrombocythemic myeloid metaplasia.

Mesa et al. [28] also wondered whether the assessment of BM angiogenesis made it possible to differentiate reactive thrombocytosis from ET. This is of particular interest given the absence of pathognomonic histological features in ET. Sensitivity and specificity of an ET histological score (0–3) based on the presence or absence of marked angiogenesis (MVG >3) and markedly decreased megakaryocyte c-Mpl (MPL) were 97 and 95% for an ET histological score cutoff set at the value of 1 or more when investi-

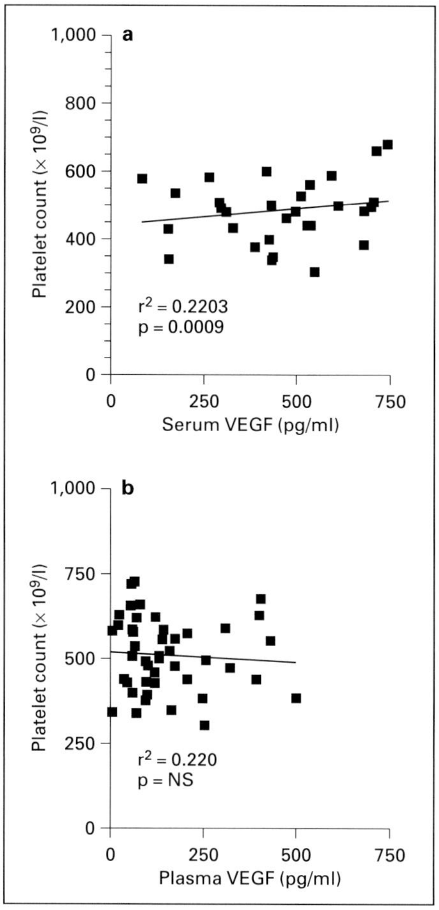

Fig. 4. Correlation between platelet count and VEGF serum (**a**) and plasma (**b**) levels.

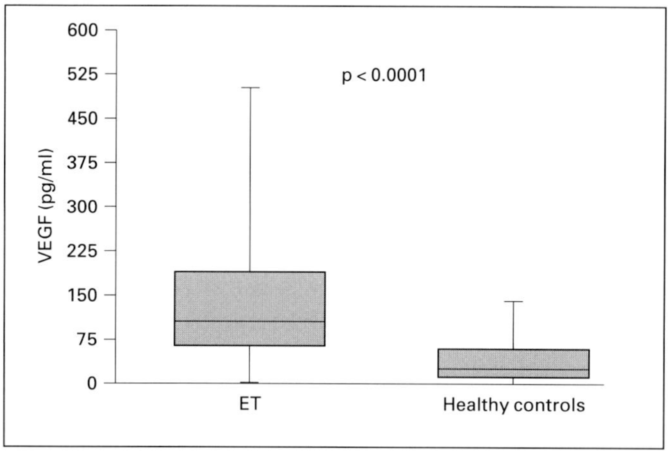

Fig. 5. VEGF plasma levels in ET patients and controls.

gators tried to distinguish ET from reactive thrombocytosis.

As stated above platelets and megakaryocytes may be a major source for VEGF in myeloproliferative disorders. In addition, VEGF mRNA is expressed by many neoplastic cells as well as by platelets, B and T lymphocytes, granulocytes and monocytes. It is possible that during the clotting process and the separation of serum, VEGF is released from platelets and other cells involved in clot formation, leading to the detection of high levels. This is reflected in the discrepancy between serum and plasma levels of VEGF reported by many investigators and some of them recommend the use of plasma rather than serum for measuring circulating angiogenic factors [29]. This issue is of particular relevance in ET. In a series of 47 ET patients in whom circulating levels of VEGF were measured in either serum or plasma using an ELISA assay, we addressed this issue. The correlation between platelet count and circulating levels of VEGF observed when dealing with serum (fig. 4a) disappeared when the VEGF determinations were performed in plasma (fig. 4b). Finally, plasma levels of VEGF were significantly higher in comparison to healthy controls (fig. 5), thus pointing out that the increase of circulating angiogenic cytokine reflects an increased angiogenesis in ET.

Studies dealing with angiogenesis in PV are mainly based on a small number of patients, so results should be considered as preliminary. On visual MVD grading, a grade 3 or 4 increase in BM angiogenesis was found in 33% of the 15 patients evaluated [6]. Similar results have been reported by Willer et al. [26] in 5 PV. However, Palmblad et al. [20] have studied 23 PV patients and found that MVD and VEGF did not differ from healthy controls.

Conclusion

Findings of microvessel BM proliferation and/or increased circulating levels of angiogenic cytokines indicate that angiogenesis is increased in myeloproliferative disorders and it may have a role in the pathophysiology of these diseases. Whether the degree of neoangiogenesis may become a marker of disease activity should be investigated in larger prospective series. By evaluating the current literature it seems that MMM might have the highest level of angiogenic activity among myeloproliferative disorders. In fact, by using a semiquantitative MVD score ranging from 1 to 4 (MVG 1 = scant vessels; MVG 2 =

moderate increase in BM angiogenesis; MVG 3 = focal areas of marked BM angiogenesis; MVG 4 = confluent increase in BM angiogenesis) Mesa et al. [27] made a comparison between ET and myelofibrosis with myeloid metaplasia (MMM) patients and found that cases scoring MVG 3–4 accounted for 17% in the former group and 73% in the latter. In addition, by comparing the results obtained in our patients affected by different myeloproliferative disorders (MMM, CML and TE), we found that MMM patients had the highest median VEGF serum concentration although the difference was statistically significant in comparison to ET only (p = 0.05).

A better knowledge of the biology of myeloproliferative diseases is an essential step for the development of new drugs and in this light several antiangiogenic drugs have been proposed to be tested in controlled trials [30]. However, it should be kept in mind that in hematological diseases it is very likely that angiogenesis factors are involved not only in an autocrine loop for hematopoietic malignant cells, but also in paracrine loops, where stromal cells, stimulated by malignant cells, produce growth factors for endothelial cells and the latter in turn produce growth factors for malignant cells [31]. Therefore, three main actors are present in this scenario of increased angiogenesis: hematopoietic malignant cells, stromal cells and endothelial cells. It is likely that the inhibition of one of them is not sufficient to eliminate the disease and future therapeutic approaches should take into account the necessity to target all three components. In addition, increased angiogenesis is only one aspect of the complex alteration in cell physiology that is responsible for the malignant growth [32] and it is possible that the efficacy of thalidomide (the only antiangiogenetic drug with a so far proven activity against hematological malignancies) is also dependent on some other mechanisms of action that are probably as important as the antiangiogenic activity.

References

1 Weidner N, Folkman J: Tumor vascularity as a prognostic factor in cancer; in De Vita VT, Hellman S, Rosenberg SA (eds): Important Advances in Oncology. Philadelphia, Lippincott-Raven, 1996, pp 167–190.

2 Perez-Atayde AR, Sallan SE, Tedrow U, Connors S, Allred E, Folkman J: Spectrum of tumor angiogenesis in the bone marrow of children with acute lymphoblastic leukemia. Am J Pathol 1997;150:815–821.

3 Vacca A, Ribatti D, Presta M, Monischetti M, Iurlaro M, Ria R, Albini A, Bussolino F, Dammacco F: Bone marrow neovascularization, plasma cell angiogenic potential, and matrix metalloproteinase-2 secretion parallel progression of human multiple myeloma. Blood 1999; 93:3064–3073.

4 Thiele J, Rompcik V, Wagner S, Fisher R: Vascular architecture and collagen type IV in primary myelofibrosis and polycythaemia vera: An immunomorphometric study on trephine biopsies of the bone marrow. Br J Haematol 1992;80:227–234.

5 Lundberg LG, Lerner R, Sundelin P, Rogers R, Folkman J, Palmblad J: Bone marrow in polycythemia vera, chronic myelocytic leukemia, and myelofibrosis has an increased vascularity. Am J Pathol 2000;157:15–19.

6 Mesa RA, Hanson CA, Rajkumar SV, Schroeder GS, Tefferi A: Evaluation and clinical correlations of microvessel density in myelofibrosis with myeloid metaplasia. Blood 2000;96: 3374–3380.

7 Barosi G: Myelofibrosis with myeloid metaplasia: Diagnostic definition and prognostic classification for clinical studies and treatment guidelines. J Clin Oncol 1999;17:2954–2970.

8 Tefferi A: Myelofibrosis with myeloid metaplasia. N Engl J Med 2000;342:1255–1265.

9 Dalley A, Smith JM, Reilly JT, Neil SM: Investigation of calmodulin and basic fibroblast growth factor (bFGF) in idiopathic myelofibrosis: Evidence for a role of extracellular calmodulin in fibroblast proliferation. Br J Haematol 1996;93:856–862.

10 Le Bousse-Kerdiles M-C, Chevillard S, Charpentier A, Romquin N, Clay D, Smadja-Joffe F, Praloran V, Dupriez B, Demory J-L, Jasmin C, Martyre MC: Differential expression of transforming growth factor-β, basic fibroblast growth factor, and their receptors in CD34+ hematopoietic progenitor cells from patients with myelofibrosis and myeloid metaplasia. Blood 1996;88:4534–4546.

11 Martyre M-C, Le Bousse-Kerdiles M-C, Romquin N, Chevillard S, Praloran V, Demory J-L, Dupriez B: Elevated levels of basic fibroblast growth factor in megakaryocytes and platelets from patients with idiopathic myelofibrosis. Br J Haematol 1997;97:441–448.

12 Vermeulen PB, Gasparini G, Fox SB, Toi M, Martin L, McCulloch P, Pezzella F, Viale G, Weidner S, Harris AL, Dirix LY: Quantification of angiogenesis in solid human tumors: An international consensus on the methodology and criteria of evaluation. Eur J Cancer 1996; 32A:2474–2484.

13 Ferrara N, Davis-Smyth T: Biology of vascular endothelial growth factor. Endocr Rev 1997; 18:4–25.

14 Kim J: Inhibition of vascular endothelial growth factor-induced angiogenesis suppresses tumor growth in vitro. Nature 1993;362:841–844.

15 Di Raimondo F, Azzaro MP, Palumbo GA, Bagnato S, Stagno F, Giustolisi GM, Cacciola E, Sortino G, Guglielmo P, Giustolisi R: Elevated vascular endothelial growth factor (VEGF) serum levels in idiopathic myelofibrosis. Leukemia 2001;15:976–980.

16 Mohle R, Green D, Moore MA, Nachman RL, Rafii S: Constitutive production and thrombin-induced release of vascular endothelial growth factor by human megakaryocytes and platelets. Proc Natl Acad Sci USA 1997;94: 663–668.

17 Ziegler BL, Valtieri M, Almeida Porada G, De Maria R, Muller R, Masella B, Gabbianelli M, Casella I, Pelosi E, Bock T, Zanjani ED, Peschle C: KDR receptor: A key marker defining hematopoietic stem cells. Science 1999; 285:1553–1558.

18 Jiang W, Hiscox S, Matsumoto K, Nakamura T: Hepatocyte growth factor/scatter factor, its molecular, cellular and clinical implication in cancer. Crit Rev Oncol Hematol 1999;29:209–248.

19 Thomas DA, Aguayo A, Giles FJ, Albitar M, O'Brien S, Cortes J, Faderl S, Bivins C, Zeldis J, Keating MJ, Barlogie B, Kantarjian MJ: Thalidomide anti-angiogenesis therapy (RX) in Philadelphia (Ph)-negative myeloproliferative disorders (MPD) and myelofibrosis (MF). Blood 1999;94(suppl 1):702a.

20 Palmblad J, Lerner R, Lundberg LG: Vascular density, intracellular VEGF and bFGF positivity as prognostic factors in polycythemia vera and chronic myelocytic leukemia. Blood 2000; 96(suppl 1):257b.

21 Aguayo A, Kantarjian H, Manshouri T, Gidel C, Estey E, Thomas D, Koller C, Estrov Z, O'Brian S, Keating M, Freireich E, Albitar M: Angiogenesis in acute and chronic leukemias and myelodysplastic syndromes. Blood 2000; 96:2240–2245.
22 Ratajczak MZ, Ratajczak J, Machalinski B, Majka M, Marlicz W, Carter A, Pietrzkowski Z, Gewirtz AM: Role of vascular endothelial growth factor (VEGF) and placenta-derived growth factor (PLGF) in regulating human haemopoietic cell growth. Br J Haematol 1998; 103:969–979.
23 Janowska-Wieczorek A, Majka M, Pear W, Gewirtz AM, Ratajczak MZ: Chronic myelogenous leukemia (CML) cells stimulate angiogenesis. Blood 2000;96(suppl 1):739a.
24 Di Raimondo F, Fichera E, Azzaro MP, Stagno F, Palumbo GA, Giustolisi R: Low serum levels of vascular endothelial growth factor (VEGF) and hepatocyte growth factor (HGF) in IFN-treated chronic myeloid leukemia (CML) patients. Blood 2000;96(suppl 1):253b.
25 Di Raimondo F, Palumbo GA, Azzaro MP, Giustolisi R: Angiogenesis in acute myeloid leukemia. Blood 2000;96:3656–3659.
26 Willer A, Hastka J, La Rosee P, Saussele S, Reiter A, Kuhn C, Hochaus A, Hehlmann R: Angiogenesis in chronic myeloproliferative disorders. Blood 2000;96(suppl 1):748a.
27 Mesa RA, Hanson CA, Li CY, Yoon SY, Schroeder GS, Tefferi A: Bone marrow immunohistochemical features complement histology in distinguishing essential thrombocythemia from reactive thrombocytosis (abstract). Blood 2000;96(suppl 1):3214.
28 Mesa RA, Li CY, Yoon SY, Schroeder GS, Tefferi A: Clinical correlates of megakaryocyte c-mpl expression in essential thrombocythemia: A clinicopathologic study of 169 patients (abstract). Blood 2000;96(suppl 1):3208.
29 Wynendaele W, Derua R, Hoylaerts MF, Pawinski A, Waelkens E, de Bruijn EA, Paridaens R, Merlevede W, van Oosterom AT: Vascular endothelial growth factor measured in platelet poor plasma allows optimal separation between cancer patients and volunteers: A key to study an angiogenic marker in vivo? Ann Oncol 1999;10:965–971.
30 Talks KL, Harris AL: Current status of antiangiogenic factors. Br J Haematol 2000;109:477–489.
31 Bertolini F, Mancuso P, Gobbi A, Pruneri G: The thin red line: Angiogenesis in normal and malignant hematopoiesis. Exp Hematol 2000; 28:993–1000.
32 Hanahan D, Weinberg RA: The hallmarks of cancer. Cell 2000;100:57–70.

Acta Haematologica

Acta Haematol 2001;106:184–189

Angiogenesis in Lymphoproliferative Disorders

Petri Salven

Division of Hematology-Oncology, Weill Medical College of Cornell University, New York, N.Y., USA

Key Words
Angiogenesis · Fibroblast growth factor, basic · Leukemia · Lymphoma · Lymphoproliferative disorders · Malignancies, hematological · Multiple myeloma · Vascular endothelial growth factor

Abstract
In this review, the cellular and molecular mechanisms underlying angiogenesis in lymphoproliferative disorders are summarized, alongside with possible therapeutic applications. Although most of the initial studies in angiogenesis were done on solid tumors, recent data demonstrate the importance of angiogenesis in hematological malignancies including leukemia, lymphoma, and multiple myeloma. Expression of angiogenic polypeptides vascular endothelial growth factor (VEGF) and basic fibroblast growth factor (bFGF) correlate with clinical characteristics in leukemia and lymphoma, and their serum concentrations serve as predictors of poor prognosis. Antiangiogenic drugs, including thalidomide, arsenic trioxide, endostatin, vasostatin, and neutralizing antibodies to VEGF receptors, used alone or in combination with established chemo- or immunotherapy regimens, constitute a promising approach for the treatment of lymphoproliferative disorders.

Introduction

Angiogenesis, the sprouting of new capillaries from pre-existing ones, is an important component in many physiological and pathological processes. In healthy adults extensive angiogenesis occurs only in the female reproductive system [1] and during tissue repair and wound healing [2]. Under certain pathological circumstances, inhibitory controls are unable to restrain the increased activity of angiogenic inducers, and excessive angiogenesis is integral to the pathology [3, 4]. These conditions include cardiovascular diseases (atherosclerosis), chronic inflammation (rheumatoid arthritis, inflammatory bowel disease), diabetes (diabetic retinopathy), psoriasis, endometriosis, and cancer [2, 5]. Promoting the formation of new collateral vessels in ischemic tissues using angiogenic growth factors (therapeutic angiogenesis) is an exciting frontier of cardiovascular medicine. Conversely, inhibition of the action of key regulators of angiogenesis constitutes a promising approach for the treatment of cancer and intraocular neovascular syndromes [6].

Role of Angiogenesis in Lymphoproliferative Disorders

In cancer, active angiogenesis is a prerequisite for tumor growth beyond a few mm^3 in size [2]. In addition, the dissemination of malignant tumors is dependent on angiogenesis [7]. Analyses of metastatic colonies in mouse

KARGER
Fax +41 61 306 12 34
E-Mail karger@karger.ch
www.karger.com

0001–5792/01/1064–0184$17.50/0

Accessible online at:
www.karger.com/journals/aha

Petri Salven, MD, PhD
Division of Hematology-Oncology, Weill Medical College of Cornell University
1300 York Avenue, Room C-606, New York, NY 10021 (USA)
Tel. +1 212 746 2017, Fax +1 509 692 0650
E-Mail pjs2004@med.cornell.edu, petri.salven@helsinki.fi

lungs have revealed that the colonies must become neovascularized before they can grow larger than microscopic in size [8, 9]. It has been shown that solid tumors progress in concert with an induction of tumor angiogenesis. Although most of the initial studies in angiogenesis were done on solid tumors, there are data suggesting the importance of angiogenesis in hematological malignancies. Already in 1975, Wolf and Hubler [10] described a subcutaneous lymphoma mimicking a vascular neoplasm because of the extensive telangiectasia overlying the tumor. Fragments of the lymphoma inserted in the hamster cheek pouch membrane induced dramatic neovascularization making the authors suggest that a diffusible tumor angiogenic factor may play a vital role. More recent data demonstrate that when bone marrow biopsies from children with newly diagnosed, untreated acute lymphoblastic leukemia and from controls are evaluated, the biopsies from children with leukemia show significantly higher microvessel densities. This suggests that leukemia cells induce angiogenesis in the bone marrow and that leukemia might be angiogenesis dependent [11]. In agreement, the microvessel densities in bone marrow samples from patients with acute myeloid leukemia (AML) are significantly higher than those in normal marrows [12, 13]. In a series of 145 patients, except for chronic lymphocytic leukemia (CLL), bone marrow vascularity was significantly higher in all leukemias and myelodysplastic syndromes compared with control bone marrows. The highest number of blood vessels and largest vascular area were found in chronic myeloid leukemia [14]. Similarly, in non-Hodgkin's lymphomas (NHL), significantly higher microvessel counts are found in high-grade lymphomas than in low-grade lymphomas, implying that angiogenesis occurring in NHLs increases with tumor progression [15, 16]. The extent of angiogenesis, measured by microvessel counts, increases simultaneously with pathological progression in B cell NHL [16]. Microvessel density also discriminates between cutaneous B cell lymphomas and B cell pseudolymphomas [17]. Recently, angiogenesis was shown to be an early event in the generation of myc-induced lymphomas [18]. Elevated microvessel densities of bone marrow have also been observed in myelodysplastic syndromes [19]. A high correlation between the extent of bone marrow angiogenesis, evaluated as microvessel area, and the proliferating (S phase) fraction of marrow plasma cells has been found in patients with multiple myeloma (MM) and in those with monoclonal gammopathies of undetermined significance. In the same study, angiogenesis itself was significantly associated with active as opposed to nonactive MM and monoclonal gammopathies of undetermined significance, and the highest microvessel area accompanied rapidly progressive MM [20]. In line, the bone marrow microvessel area has been observed to increase simultaneously with the progression of MM [21], and bone marrow angiogenesis, assessed by counting the microvessel density, has been shown to be a predictor of poor survival in newly diagnosed MM [22]. Interestingly, bone marrow neovascularization has been described to be particularly high in MM with the deletion of chromosome 13q [23].

Angiogenic Molecules in Lymphoproliferative Disorders

Angiogenesis is considered to depend on the balance of inhibitors and stimulators of endothelial cell proliferation, endothelial cell migration, and capillary formation molecules [3, 4, 24]. The constantly growing list of angiogenic molecules includes angiopoietin-1, angiotropin, angiogenin, basic fibroblast growth factor (bFGF), erythropoietin, vascular endothelial growth factor (VEGF), VEGF-B, VEGF-C, interleukins, hormones and chemokines. VEGF, also called vascular permeability factor (VPF) [25, 26], and bFGF, also called fibroblast growth factor-2 (FGF-2) [27, 28], are often thought to play central roles in the regulation of angiogenesis. VEGF and bFGF are secreted multifunctional cytokines that are mitogens for endothelial cells and potent inducers of angiogenesis in vivo. Expression of VEGF in tumor xenografts in nude mice has been shown to enhance tumor growth and tumor angiogenesis [29, 30]. In a transgenic mouse model the angiogenic switch in bovine papilloma virus-induced fibrosarcoma correlates with the export of bFGF from cells [31]. The important role of these angiogenic factors has been shown in vivo by immunoneutralizing antibodies against VEGF [32–34] or bFGF [35], which inhibit tumor growth in nude mice.

VEGF derives from cancer cells themselves [36, 37], and other cells at the site, including circulating and tissue infiltrating inflammatory cells [38–40]. Blood cells including peripheral blood mononuclear cells (PBMNCs) [40], T cells [38, 41], B cells [41], neutrophils [42], and platelets [40, 43, 44] contain and transport VEGF. Whole blood from patients with disseminated lymphoma contains significantly elevated levels of VEGF [40]. Circulating levels of VEGF have been shown to correlate with overall survival [45, 46] and event-free survival [47] in NHL, and with progression-free survival in CLL [48]. Expression of angiogenic molecules including VEGF and VEGF-C has been observed in tumor tissue samples from patients with lymphoma [49, 50]. A significant expression of VEGF transcripts was also observed in Hodgkin's disease and peripheral T cell lymphomas, particularly of the angioimmunoblastic type [51]. In contrast, in normal and ulcerated tonsils, VEGF was expressed in the squamous epithelium but only rarely found in the lymphoid tissue. [51]. VEGF transcription was observed in 23 of 33 (69%) of patients with AML [52]. In addition, an increased cellular VEGF content is a predictor of unfavorable outcome in patients with AML [53]. VEGF is expressed and secreted by myeloma cell lines and plasma cells isolated from bone marrow of patients with MM [54]. Also in multicentric Castleman's disease, an atypical lymphoproliferative disorder thought to be related to immune dysregulation [55], lymphoid hyperplasia is often associated with evidence of excessive vascularization in the germinal centers that has been attributed to local VEGF expression [51].

VEGF may also have autocrine potential in leukemia and lymphoma. When human hematopoietic tumor cell lines, representing multiple lineages and diseases, including leukemia, lymphoma, and MM were studied, results revealed that the VEGF message was expressed in these cells and that the corresponding protein was secreted into the extracellular environment. Interestingly, 5 of the 12 cell lines studied were also found to express VEGF receptor 1 (VEGFR-1) at a moderate to strong level, suggesting an autocrine pathway [56]. Similarly, certain leukemias not only produce VEGF but also express functional VEGFR-2 in vivo and in vitro, resulting in the generation of an autocrine loop that may support leukemic cell survival and proliferation. Approximately 50% of freshly isolated leukemias expressed mRNA and protein for VEGFR-2 [57]. In a tumor animal model using xenotransplanted human leukemia and lymphoma cell lines, a strong correlation was observed between the amount of VEGF produced in vitro by cultured cells and the efficiency of tumor engraftment [58].

Peripheral blood megakaryocytes and platelets have been shown to contain bFGF [59]. PBMNCs [60], T cells [61, 62], and granulocytes [59] have also been reported to contain bFGF mRNA or protein. Interestingly, PBMNCs derived from patients suffering from hairy cell leukemia secreted relatively high levels of bFGF in culture media while bFGF was not detectable in PBMNC cultures from healthy donors [63]. In addition, various lymphoblastoid and leukemic cell lines have been shown to secrete bFGF [64, 65]. In CLL an elevated intracellular level of bFGF correlates with the stage, and is also associated with resistance to chemotherapy [66]. In NHL, the elevated serum bFGF level at diagnosis serves as an independent predictor of poor prognosis [67]. Interestingly, the highest prognostic power was obtained when the serum concentrations of VEGF (S-VEGF) and bFGF (S-bFGF) were examined as a combination [46]. The NHL patients who at diagnosis had both S-VEGF and S-bFGF within the highest quartiles had only a 21% 5-year survival rate in contrast to 64% among the patients having both factors within the three lowest quartiles ($p < 0.0001$). A simultaneous elevation of S-VEGF and S-bFGF was associated with poor survival in different grades of NHL, as well as in the largest histological subgroup, the large cell diffuse and immunoblastic lymphomas. The patients with both S-VEGF and S-bFGF within the highest quartiles had a nearly 3 times higher relative risk of death than the rest of the patients. This relative risk was higher than the relative risks associated with any of the components of the international prognostic index in the same model. In line with this clinical observation, VEGF and bFGF have been shown to synergize using in vitro angiogenesis assays [68, 69], indicating that they can serve complementary functions.

Antiangiogenic Therapy of Lymphoproliferative Disorders

Several already available molecules with different established clinical properties exhibit also antiangiogenic potential. A classical example is thalidomide, which was originally developed as a sedative, but was later withdrawn because of its teratogenicity. In 1994, D'Amato et al. [70] reported that orally administered thalidomide is an inhibitor of angiogenesis. Experiments revealed that the antiangiogenic activity correlated with the teratogenicity but not with the sedative or the mild immunosuppressive properties of thalidomide. Recently, a number of studies have shown that thalidomide is active against advanced or relapsed MM, being able to induce marked and durable responses in some patients [71–76]. Arsenic trioxide has recently been used successfully in the treatment of patients with acute promyelocytic leukemia who relapsed after initial therapy with chemotherapy and all-trans retinoic acid [77–81]. Intriguingly, novel data suggest that arsenic trioxide induces dose- and time-dependent apoptosis of vascular endothelium, and may thus exert the antileukemic effect via inhibition of angiogenesis [82]. By using an antiangiogenic dosing schedule of cyclophosphamide that provided more sustained apoptosis of endothelial cells, Browder et al. [83] showed that a chemotherapeutic agent can effectively control leukemia growth in mice, regardless of whether the cancer cells are drug resistant. Inhibition of angiogenesis and induction of endothelial and tumor cell apoptosis in animal models of human high-grade NHL has also been achieved by green tea [84].

VEGF is such a potent and critical vascular regulator that its dosage must be exquisitely regulated to avoid vascular disaster. Disruption of even a single VEGF allele in mice leads to embryonic lethality due to severe vascular abnormalities, providing perhaps the only example of embryonic lethality due to a simple half-dosage effect [85, 86]. Therefore, inhibiting angiogenesis by interruption of signaling by VEGFRs, particularly VEGFR-2, may provide a powerful therapeutic strategy [6]. VEGF may have autocrine potential in leukemia and lymphoma [56–58], making this strategy even more attractive in hematopoietic malignancies. Indeed, injection of neutralizing antibody, specific to human VEGFR-2, was recently shown to inhibit proliferation of xenotransplanted human leukemias, and significantly increased the survival of inoculated mice [57].

Vasostatin inhibits endothelial cell growth and neovascularization, and interleukin-12 (IL-12) targets the tumor vasculature acting through interferon-γ. Individually, vasostatin and IL-12 produced distinct efficacy profiles in trials aimed at reducing tumor growth in athymic mice. When inoculated into athymic mice, vasostatin reduced the growth of human Burkitt lymphoma [87]. In combination, vasostatin and IL-12 halted the growth of human Burkitt lymphoma in athymic mice [88]. Thus, cancer therapy that combines distinct inhibitors of angiogenesis is a novel, effective strategy for the experimental treatment of cancer. In a recent study by Bertolini et al. [89], endostatin, a specific antiangiogenic drug, was shown to induce tumor stabilization after chemotherapy or anti-CD20 immunotherapy in a mouse model of human high-grade NHL. When given after chemotherapy or immunotherapy, endostatin effectively induced tumor stabilization, and tumor growth was prevented in endostatin-treated mice as long as the drug was administered. Remarkably, administration of endostatin on days 25–29 after tumor regrowth still induced significant tumor regression, whereas chemotherapy and anti-CD20 immunotherapy were not effective. Taken together, inhibition of the action of key regulators of angiogenesis, alone or in combination with other antiangiogenic drugs and/or established chemo- or immunotherapy regimens, constitutes a promising approach for the treatment of lymphoproliferative disorders.

Acknowledgements

This work was supported by grants from the Sigrid Juselius Foundation, the Finnish Medical Foundation, the Maud Kuistila Memorial Foundation, and the Ella and Georg Ehrnrooth Foundation.

References

1 Reynolds LP, Killilea SD, Redmer DA: Angiogenesis in the female reproductive system. FASEB J 1992;6:886–892.
2 Folkman J: Angiogenesis in cancer, vascular, rheumatoid and other disease. Nat Med 1995; 1:27–31.
3 Risau W: Differentiation of endothelium. FASEB J 1995;9:926–933.
4 Hanahan D, Folkman J: Patterns and emerging mechanisms of the angiogenic switch during tumorigenesis. Cell 1996;86:353–364.
5 Griffioen AW, Molema G: Angiogenesis: Potential for pharmacologic intervention in the treatment of cancer, cardiovascular diseases, and chronic inflammation. Pharmacol Rev 2000;52:238–262.
6 Ferrara N, Alitalo K: Clinical applications of angiogenic growth factors and their inhibitors. Nat Med 1999;5:1359–1364.
7 Liotta LA, Kleinerman J, Saidel GM: Quantitative relationships of intravascular tumor cells, tumor vessels, and pulmonary metastases following tumor implantation. Cancer Res 1974;34:997–1004.
8 O'Reilly MS, Holmgren L, Shing Y, Chen C, Rosenthal RA, Moses M, Lane WS, Cao Y, Sage EH, Folkman J: Angiostatin: A novel angiogenesis inhibitor that mediates the suppression of metastases by a Lewis lung carcinoma. Cell 1994;79:315–328.
9 Holmgren L, O'Reilly MS, Folkman J: Dormancy of micrometastases: Balanced proliferation and apoptosis in the presence of angiogenesis suppression. Nat Med 1995;1:149–153.
10 Wolf JE, Hubler WR: Tumour angiogenic factor associated with subcutaneous lymphoma. Br J Dermatol 1975;92:273–277.
11 Perez-Atayde AR, Sallan SE, Tedrow U, Connors S, Allred E, Folkman J: Spectrum of tumor angiogenesis in the bone marrow of children with acute lymphoblastic leukemia. Am J Pathol 1997;150:815–821.
12 Hussong JW, Rodgers GM, Shami PJ: Evidence of increased angiogenesis in patients with acute myeloid leukemia. Blood 2000;95: 309–313.
13 Padro T, Ruiz S, Bieker R, Burger H, Steins M, Kienast J, Buchner T, Berdel WE, Mesters RM: Increased angiogenesis in the bone marrow of patients with acute myeloid leukemia. Blood 2000;95:2637–2644.
14 Aguayo A, Kantarjian H, Manshouri T, Gidel C, Estey E, Thomas D, Koller C, Estrov Z, O'Brien S, Keating M, Freireich E, Albitar M: Angiogenesis in acute and chronic leukemias and myelodysplastic syndromes. Blood 2000; 96:2240–2245.
15 Ribatti D, Vacca A, Nico B, Fanelli M, Roncali L, Dammacco F: Angiogenesis spectrum in the stroma of B-cell non-Hodgkin's lymphomas. An immunohistochemical and ultrastructural study. Eur J Haematol 1996;56:45–53.
16 Vacca A, Ribatti D, Ruco L, Giacchetta F, Nico B, Quondamatteo F, Ria R, Iurlaro M, Dammacco F: Angiogenesis extent and macrophage density increase simultaneously with pathological progression in B-cell non-Hodgkin's lymphomas. Br J Cancer 1999;79:965–970.

17 Schaerer L, Schmid MH, Mueller B, Dummer RG, Burg G, Kempf W: Angiogenesis in cutaneous lymphoproliferative disorders: Microvessel density discriminates between cutaneous B-cell lymphomas and B-cell pseudolymphomas. Am J Dermatopathol 2000;22:140–143.
18 Brandvold KA, Neiman P, Ruddell A: Angiogenesis is an early event in the generation of myc-induced lymphomas. Oncogene 2000;19: 2780–2785.
19 Pruneri G, Bertolini F, Soligo D, Carboni N, Cortelezzi A, Ferrucci PF, Buffa R, Lambertenghi-Deliliers G, Pezzella F: Angiogenesis in myelodysplastic syndromes. Br J Cancer 1999; 81:1398–1401.
20 Vacca A, Ribatti D, Roncali L, Ranieri G, Serio G, Silvestris F, Dammacco F: Bone marrow angiogenesis and progression in multiple myeloma. Br J Haematol 1994;87:503–508.
21 Ribatti D, Vacca A, Nico B, Quondamatteo F, Ria R, Minischetti M, Marzullo A, Herken R, Roncali L, Dammacco F: Bone marrow angiogenesis and mast cell density increase simultaneously with progression of human multiple myeloma. Br J Cancer 1999;79:451–455.
22 Rajkumar SV, Leong T, Roche PC, Fonseca R, Dispenzieri A, Lacy MQ, Lust JA, Witzig TE, Kyle RA, Gertz MA, Greipp PR: Prognostic value of bone marrow angiogenesis in multiple myeloma. Clin Cancer Res 2000;6:3111–3116.
23 Schreiber S, Ackermann J, Obermair A, Kaufmann H, Urbauer E, Aletaha K, Gisslinger H, Chott A, Huber H, Drach J: Multiple myeloma with deletion of chromosome 13q is characterized by increased bone marrow neovascularization. Br J Haematol 2000;110:605–609.
24 Yancopoulos GD, Davis S, Gale NW, Rudge JS, Wiegand SJ, Holash J: Vascular-specific growth factors and blood vessel formation. Nature 2000;407:242–248.
25 Dvorak HF, Brown LF, Detmar M, Dvorak AM: Vascular permeability factor/vascular endothelial growth factor, microvascular hyperpermeability, and angiogenesis. Am J Pathol 1995;146:1029–1039.
26 Ferrara N, Davis-Smyth T: The biology of vascular endothelial growth factor. Endocr Rev 1997;18:4–25.
27 Friesel RE, Maciag T: Molecular mechanisms of angiogenesis: Fibroblast growth factor signal transduction. FASEB J 1995;9:919–925.
28 Bikfalvi A, Klein S, Pintucci G, Rifkin DB: Biological roles of fibroblast growth factor-2. Endocr Rev 1997;18:26–45.
29 Ferrara N, Winer J, Burton T, Rowland A, Siegel M, Phillips HS, Terrell T, Keller GA, Levinson AD: Expression of vascular endothelial growth factor does not promote transformation but confers a growth advantage in vivo to Chinese hamster ovary cells. J Clin Invest 1993;91: 160–170.
30 Zhang HT, Craft P, Scott PA, Ziche M, Weich HA, Harris AL, Bicknell R: Enhancement of tumor growth and vascular density by transfection of vascular endothelial cell growth factor into MCF-7 human breast carcinoma cells. J Natl Cancer Inst 1995;87:213–219.
31 Kandel J, Bossy-Wetzel E, Radvanyi F, Klagsbrun M, Folkman J, Hanahan D: Neovascularization is associated with a switch to the export of bFGF in the multistep development of fibrosarcoma. Cell 1991;66:1095–1104.
32 Kim KJ, Li B, Winer J, Armanini M, Gillett N, Phillips HS, Ferrara N: Inhibition of vascular endothelial growth factor-induced angiogenesis suppresses tumour growth in vivo. Nature 1993;362:841–844.
33 Asano M, Yukita A, Matsumoto T, Kondo S, Suzuki H: Inhibition of tumor growth and metastasis by an immunoneutralizing monoclonal antibody to human vascular endothelial growth factor/vascular permeability factor 121. Cancer Res 1995;55:5296–5301.
34 Warren RS, Yuan H, Matli MR, Gillett NA, Ferrara N: Regulation by vascular endothelial growth factor of human colon cancer tumorigenesis in a mouse model of experimental liver metastasis. J Clin Invest 1995;95:1789–1797.
35 Hori A, Sasada R, Matsutani E, Naito K, Sakura Y, Fujita T, Kozai Y: Suppression of solid tumor growth by immunoneutralizing monoclonal antibody against human basic fibroblast growth factor. Cancer Res 1991;51:6180–6184.
36 Neufeld G, Cohen T, Gengrinovitch S, Poltorak Z: Vascular endothelial growth factor (VEGF) and its receptors. FASEB J 1999;13: 9–22.
37 Veikkola T, Karkkainen M, Claesson-Welsh L, Alitalo K: Regulation of angiogenesis via vascular endothelial growth factor receptors. Cancer Res 2000;60:203–212.
38 Freeman MR, Schneck FX, Gagnon ML, Corless C, Soker S, Niknejad K, Peoples GE, Klagsbrun M: Peripheral blood T lymphocytes and lymphocytes infiltrating human cancers express vascular endothelial growth factor: A potential role for T cells in angiogenesis. Cancer Res 1995;55:4140–4145.
39 Salven P, Heikkila P, Anttonen A, Kajanti M, Joensuu H: Vascular endothelial growth factor in squamous cell head and neck carcinoma: Expression and prognostic significance. Mod Pathol 1997;10:1128–1133.
40 Salven P, Orpana A, Joensuu H: Leukocytes and platelets of patients with cancer contain high levels of vascular endothelial growth factor. Clin Cancer Res 1999;5:487–491.
41 Salven P, Anttonen K, Repo H, Joensuu H, Orpana A: Endotoxins induce and interferon-α suppresses VEGF production in human peripheral blood mononuclear cells. FASEB J 2001;10.1096/fj.00-0627fje.
42 Gaudry M, Bregerie O, Andrieu V, El Benna J, Pocidalo MA, Hakim J: Intracellular pool of vascular endothelial growth factor in human neutrophils. Blood 1997;90:4153–4161.
43 Mohle R, Green D, Moore MA, Nachman RL, Rafii S: Constitutive production and thrombin-induced release of vascular endothelial growth factor by human megakaryocytes and platelets. Proc Natl Acad Sci USA 1997;94: 663–668.
44 Wartiovaara U, Salven P, Mikkola H, Lassila R, Kaukonen J, Joukov V, Orpana A, Ristimaki A, Heikinheimo M, Joensuu H, Alitalo K, Palotie A: Peripheral blood platelets express VEGF-C and VEGF which are released during platelet activation. Thromb Haemost 1998;80: 171–175.
45 Salven P, Teerenhovi L, Joensuu H: A high pretreatment serum vascular endothelial growth factor concentration is associated with poor outcome in non-Hodgkin's lymphoma. Blood 1997;90:3167–3172.
46 Salven P, Orpana A, Teerenhovi L, Joensuu H: Simultaneous elevation in the serum concentrations of the angiogenic growth factors VEGF and bFGF is an independent predictor of poor prognosis in non-Hodgkin lymphoma: A single-institution study of 200 patients. Blood 2000; 96:3712–3718.
47 Bertolini F, Paolucci M, Peccatori F, Cinieri S, Agazzi A, Ferrucci PF, Cocorocchio E, Goldhirsch A, Martinelli G: Angiogenic growth factors and endostatin in non-Hodgkin's lymphoma. Br J Haematol 1999;106:504–509.
48 Molica S, Vitelli G, Levato D, Gandolfo GM, Liso V: Increased serum levels of vascular endothelial growth factor predict risk of progression in early B-cell chronic lymphocytic leukaemia. Br J Haematol 1999;107:605–610.
49 Dvorak HF, Sioussat TM, Brown LF, Berse B, Nagy JA, Sotrel A, Manseau EJ, Van de Water L, Senger DR: Distribution of vascular permeability factor (vascular endothelial growth factor) in tumors: Concentration in tumor blood vessels. J Exp Med 1991;174:1275–1278.
50 Salven P, Lymboussaki A, Heikkila P, Jaaskela-Saari H, Enholm B, Aase K, von Euler G, Eriksson U, Alitalo K, Joensuu H: Vascular endothelial growth factors VEGF-B and VEGF-C are expressed in human tumors. Am J Pathol 1998;153:103–108.
51 Foss HD, Araujo I, Demel G, Klotzbach H, Hummel M, Stein H: Expression of vascular endothelial growth factor in lymphomas and Castleman's disease. J Pathol 1997;183:44–50.
52 Fiedler W, Graeven U, Ergün S, Verago S, Kilic N, Stockschläder M, Hossfeld DK: Vascular endothelial growth factor, a possible paracrine in human acute myeloid leukemias. Blood 1997;89:1870–1875.
53 Aguayo A, Estey E, Kantarjian H, Mansouri T, Gidel C, Keating M, Giles F, Estrov Z, Barlogie B, Albitar M: Cellular vascular endothelial growth factor is a predictor of outcome in patients with acute myeloid leukemia. Blood 1999;94:3717–3721.
54 Dankbar B, Padro T, Leo R, Feldmann B, Kropff M, Mesters RM, Serve H, Berdel WE, Kienast J: Vascular endothelial growth factor and interleukin-6 in paracrine tumor-stromal cell interactions in multiple myeloma. Blood 2000;95:2630–2636.
55 Frizzera G: Atypical lymphoproliferative disorders; in Knowles DM (ed): Neoplastic Hematopathology. Baltimore, Williams & Wilkins, 2000, pp 459–496.
56 Bellamy WT, Richter L, Frutiger Y, Grogan TM: Expression of vascular endothelial growth factor and its receptors in hematopoietic malignancies. Cancer Res 1999;59:728–733.

57 Dias S, Hattori K, Zhu Z, Heissig B, Choy M, Lane W, Wu Y, Chadburn A, Hyjek E, Gill M, Hicklin DJ, Witte L, Moore MA, Rafii S: Autocrine stimulation of VEGFR-2 activates human leukemic cell growth and migration. J Clin Invest 2000;106:511–521.
58 Fusetti L, Pruneri G, Gobbi A, Rabascio C, Carboni N, Peccatori F, Martinelli G, Bertolini F: Human myeloid and lymphoid malignancies in the non-obese diabetic/severe combined immunodeficiency mouse model: Frequency of apoptotic cells in solid tumors and efficiency and speed of engraftment correlate with vascular endothelial growth factor production. Cancer Res 2000;60:2527–2534.
59 Brunner G, Nguyen H, Gabrilove J, Rifkin DB, Wilson EL: Basic fibroblast growth factor expression in human bone marrow and peripheral blood cells. Blood 1993;81:631–638.
60 Gu XF, Bikfalvi A, Chen YZ, Caen JP, Han ZC: Constitutive and selective expression of basic fibroblast growth factor in human leukaemia cell lines. Eur J Haematol 1995;55: 189–194.
61 Peoples GE, Blotnick S, Takahashi K, Freeman MR, Klagsbrun M, Eberlein TJ: T lymphocytes that infiltrate tumors and atherosclerotic plaques produce heparin-binding epidermal growth factor-like growth factor and basic fibroblast growth factor: A potential pathologic role. Proc Natl Acad Sci USA 1995;92:6547–6551.
62 Blotnick S, Peoples GE, Freeman MR, Eberlein TJ, Klagsbrun M: T lymphocytes synthesize and export heparin-binding epidermal growth factor-like growth factor and basic fibroblast growth factor, mitogens for vascular cells and fibroblasts: Differential production and release by CD4+ and CD8+ T cells. Proc Natl Acad Sci USA 1994;91:2890–2894.
63 Gruber G, Schwarzmeier JD, Shehata M, Hilgarth M, Berger R: Basic fibroblast growth factor is expressed by CD19/CD11c-positive cells in hairy cell leukemia. Blood 1999;94:1077–1085.
64 Vacca A, Ribatti D, Iurlaro M, Albini A, Minischetti M, Bussolino F, Pellegrino A, Ria R, Rusnati M, Presta M, Vincenti V, Persico MG, Dammacco F: Human lymphoblastoid cells produce extracellular matrix-degrading enzymes and induce endothelial cell proliferation, migration, morphogenesis, and angiogenesis. Int J Clin Lab Res 1998;28:55–68.
65 Allouche M, Bayard F, Clamens S, Fillola G, Sie P, Amalric F: Expression of basic fibroblast growth factor (bFGF) and FGF-receptors in human leukemic cells. Leukemia 1995;9:77–86.
66 Menzel T, Rahman Z, Calleja E, White K, Wilson EL, Wieder R, Gabrilove J: Elevated intracellular level of basic fibroblast growth factor correlates with stage of chronic lymphocytic leukemia and is associated with resistance to fludarabine. Blood 1996;87:1056–1063.
67 Salven P, Teerenhovi L, Joensuu H: A high pretreatment serum basic fibroblast growth factor concentration is an independent predictor of poor prognosis in non-Hodgkin's lymphoma. Blood 1999;94:3334–3339.
68 Pepper MS, Ferrara N, Orci L, Montesano R: Potent synergism between vascular endothelial growth factor and basic fibroblast growth factor in the induction of angiogenesis in vitro. Biochem Biophys Res Commun 1992;189:824–831.
69 Goto F, Goto K, Weindel K, Folkman J: Synergistic effects of vascular endothelial growth factor and basic fibroblast growth factor on the proliferation and cord formation of bovine capillary endothelial cells within collagen gels. Lab Invest 1993;69:508–517.
70 D'Amato RJ, Loughnan MS, Flynn E, Folkman J: Thalidomide is an inhibitor of angiogenesis. Proc Natl Acad Sci USA 1994;91: 4082–4085.
71 Singhal S, Mehta J, Desikan R, Ayers D, Roberson P, Eddlemon P, Munshi N, Anaissie E, Wilson C, Dhodapkar M, Zeddis J, Barlogie B: Antitumor activity of thalidomide in refractory multiple myeloma. N Engl J Med 1999;341: 1565–1571.
72 Hideshima T, Chauhan D, Shima Y, Raje N, Davies FE, Tai YT, Treon SP, Lin B, Schlossman RL, Richardson P, Muller G, Stirling DI, Anderson KC: Thalidomide and its analogs overcome drug resistance of human multiple myeloma cells to conventional therapy. Blood 2000;96:2943–2950.
73 Zomas A, Anagnostopoulos N, Dimopoulos MA: Successful treatment of multiple myeloma relapsing after high-dose therapy and autologous transplantation with thalidomide as a single agent. Bone Marrow Transplant 2000;25: 1319–1320.
74 Juliusson G, Celsing F, Turesson I, Lenhoff S, Adriansson M, Malm C: Frequent good partial remissions from thalidomide including best response ever in patients with advanced refractory and relapsed myeloma. Br J Haematol 2000; 109:89–96.
75 Kneller A, Raanani P, Hardan I, Avigdor A, Levi I, Berkowicz M, Ben-Bassat I: Therapy with thalidomide in refractory multiple myeloma patients – The revival of an old drug. Br J Haematol 2000;108:391–393.
76 Rajkumar SV, Fonseca R, Dispenzieri A, Lacy MQ, Lust JA, Witzig TE, Kyle RA, Gertz MA, Greipp PR: Thalidomide in the treatment of relapsed multiple myeloma. Mayo Clin Proc 2000;75:897–901.
77 Shen ZX, Chen GQ, Ni JH, Li XS, Xiong SM, Qiu QY, Zhu J, Tang W, Sun GL, Yang KQ, Chen Y, Zhou L, Fang ZW, Wang YT, Ma J, Zhang P, Zhang TD, Chen SJ, Chen Z, Wang ZY: Use of arsenic trioxide (As_2O_3) in the treatment of acute promyelocytic leukemia (APL). II. Clinical efficacy and pharmacokinetics in relapsed patients. Blood 1997;89:3354–3360.
78 Soignet SL, Maslak P, Wang ZG, Jhanwar S, Calleja E, Dardashti LJ, Corso D, DeBlasio A, Gabrilove J, Scheinberg DA, Pandolfi PP, Warrell RP Jr: Complete remission after treatment of acute promyelocytic leukemia with arsenic trioxide. N Engl J Med 1998;339:1341–1348.
79 Agis H, Weltermann A, Mitterbauer G, Thalhammer R, Edelhauser M, Seewann HL, Valent P, Lechner K, Fonatsch C, Geissler K: Successful treatment with arsenic trioxide of a patient with ATRA-resistant relapse of acute promyelocytic leukemia. Ann Hematol 1999; 78:329–332.
80 Galimberti S, Papineschi F, Carmignani A, Testi R, Fazzi R, Petrini M: Arsenic and all-trans retinoic acid as induction therapy before autograft in a case of relapsed resistant secondary acute promyelocytic leukemia. Bone Marrow Transplant 1999;24:345–348.
81 Niu C, Yan H, Yu T, Sun HP, Liu JX, Li XS, Wu W, Zhang FQ, Chen Y, Zhou L, Li JM, Zeng XY, Yang RR, Yuan MM, Ren MY, Gu FY, Cao Q, Gu BW, Su XY, Chen GQ, Xiong SM, Zhang T, Waxman S, Wang ZY, Chen SJ, et al: Studies on treatment of acute promyelocytic leukemia with arsenic trioxide: Remission induction, follow-up, and molecular monitoring in 11 newly diagnosed and 47 relapsed acute promyelocytic leukemia patients. Blood 1999;94:3315–3324.
82 Roboz GJ, Dias S, Lam G, Lane WJ, Soignet SL, Warrell RP Jr, Rafii S: Arsenic trioxide induces dose- and time-dependent apoptosis of endothelium and may exert an antileukemic effect via inhibition of angiogenesis. Blood 2000;96:1525–1530.
83 Browder T, Butterfield CE, Kraling BM, Shi B, Marshall B, O'Reilly MS, Folkman J: Antiangiogenic scheduling of chemotherapy improves efficacy against experimental drug-resistant cancer. Cancer Res 2000;60:1878–1886.
84 Bertolini F, Fusetti L, Rabascio C, Cinieri S, Martinelli G, Pruneri G: Inhibition of angiogenesis and induction of endothelial and tumor cell apoptosis by green tea in animal models of human high-grade non-Hodgkin's lymphoma. Leukemia 2000;14:1477–1482.
85 Ferrara N, Carver Moore K, Chen H, Dowd M, Lu L, O'Shea KS, Powell Braxton L, Hillan KJ, Moore MW: Heterozygous embryonic lethality induced by targeted inactivation of the VEGF gene. Nature 1996;380:439–442.
86 Carmeliet P, Ferreira V, Breier G, Pollefeyt S, Kieckens L, Gertsenstein M, Fahrig M, Vandenhoeck A, Harpal K, Eberhardt C, Declercq C, Pawling J, Moons L, Collen D, Risau W, Nagy A: Abnormal blood vessel development and lethality in embryos lacking a single VEGF allele. Nature 1996;380:435–439.
87 Pike SE, Yao L, Jones KD, Cherney B, Appella E, Sakaguchi K, Nakhasi H, Teruya-Feldstein J, Wirth P, Gupta G, Tosato G: Vasostatin, a calreticulin fragment, inhibits angiogenesis and suppresses tumor growth. J Exp Med 1998;188: 2349–2356.
88 Yao L, Pike SE, Setsuda J, Parekh J, Gupta G, Raffeld M, Jaffe ES, Tosato G: Effective targeting of tumor vasculature by the angiogenesis inhibitors vasostatin and interleukin-12. Blood 2000;96:1900–1905.
89 Bertolini F, Fusetti L, Mancuso P, Gobbi A, Corsini C, Ferrucci PF, Martinelli G, Pruneri G: Endostatin, an antiangiogenic drug, induces tumor stabilization after chemotherapy or anti-CD20 therapy in a NOD/SCID mouse model of human high-grade non-Hodgkin lymphoma. Blood 2000;96:282–287.

Acta Hæmatologica

Acta Haematol 2001;106:190–207

Antiangiogenic Therapy in Leukemia

Deborah A. Thomas Francis J. Giles Jorge Cortes Maher Albitar
Hagop M. Kantarjian

Department of Leukemia, M.D. Anderson Cancer Center, Houston, Tex., USA

Key Words
Angiogenesis · Leukemia · Vascular endothelial growth factor

Abstract
Angiogenesis is a fundamental element of the physiological processes of embryogenesis and wound healing. During malignant transformation, dysregulation of angiogenesis leads to the formation of a vascular network of tumor-associated capillaries promoting survival and proliferation of the cancerous cells. Activation, migration, proliferation and differentiation of endothelial cells into mature blood vessels is driven by several cytokines and growth factors, known to be dysregulated in hematological malignancies. Thus, therapeutic interventions designed to eradicate the malignant clone should incorporate modulation of the angiogenic cascade. Antiangiogenic agents which target different components of the neovascularization process are being investigated in various solid tumors known to have increased vascularity. The role of angiogenesis in hematological malignancies, the rationale for the use of angiosuppressive therapy for these entities, and the status of novel antiangiogenic agents in clinical trials are discussed.

Introduction

In the early 1970s, the relevance of tumor-associated angiogenesis was recognized. The fundamental elements of neovascularization and the mechanisms by which tumor cells invade and metastasize have been further characterized, particularly for solid tumor malignancies. With the development of targeted therapies, the influence of angiogenesis on clonal proliferation and prognosis in various leukemias and other hematological disorders has been explored.

Angiogenesis: Role in Clonal Proliferation

In 1971, Folkman [1] determined that angiogenesis (the development of capillaries from established blood vessels) was essential for tumor development beyond 2–3 mm in size. Tumor dormancy resulted once the clone proliferated to the capacity of normal host blood vessels. Tumors able to induce angiogenesis in surrounding host tissues were more likely to proliferate rapidly and metastasize [2–6]. In most instances, neoplastic proliferation stems first from transformation of a cell to a malignant clone, after the activation of oncogenes or inactivation (or deletion) of tumor-suppressor genes such as p53 [7]. The presence of mutant p53 correlates with increased angiogenesis [via increased vascular endothelial growth factor (VEGF) secretion] and malignant progression [7]. De-

KARGER

Fax + 41 61 306 12 34
E-Mail karger@karger.ch
www.karger.com

0001–5792/01/1064–0190$17.50/0

Accessible online at:
www.karger.com/journals/aha

Deborah A. Thomas, MD, Assistant Professor
Department of Leukemia, M.D. Anderson Cancer Center
1515 Holcombe Blvd, Box 428, Houston, TX 77030 (USA)
Tel. +1 713 745 4616, Fax +1 713 745 4612 or 794 4297
E-Mail debthomas@mdanderson.org

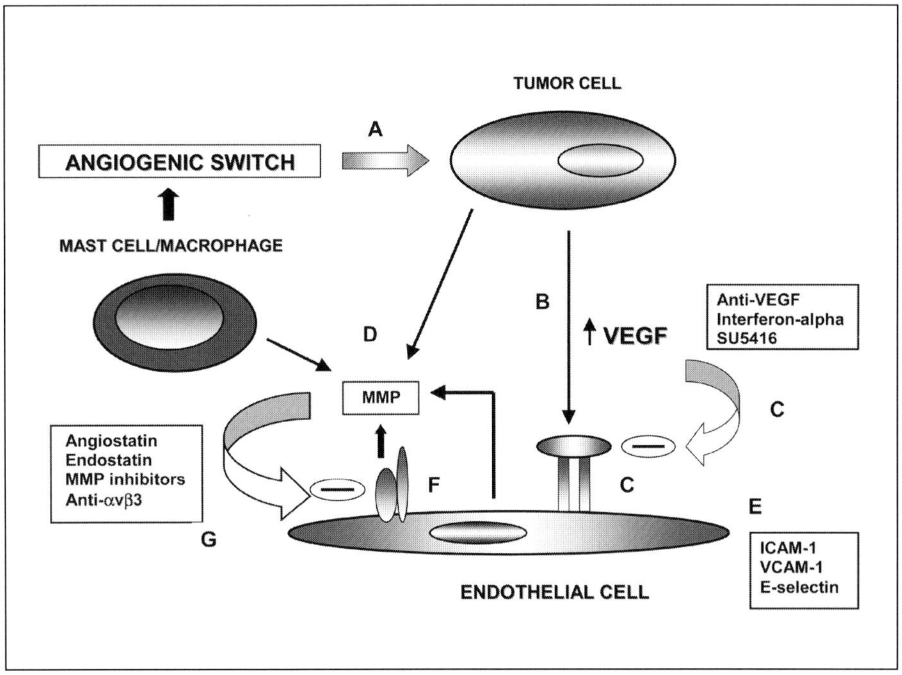

Fig. 1. A = Angiogenic 'switch' mediated by overexpression of angiogenic factors, recruitment of macrophages to produce angiogenic factors, or mobilization of angiogenic proteins from ECM results in the ability of tumor cells to stimulate neovascularization; B = VEGF binds to VEGFR on the surface of endothelial cells, leading to their activation; C = monoclonal antibodies to VEGF, tyrosine kinase inhibitors (SU5416), and IFN-α interfere with VEGF-mediated stimulation of endothelial cells; D = secretion of MMP results in degradation of the ECM, allowing invasion and migration; E = activated endothelial cells upregulate genes of adhesion molecules such as intercellular adhesion molecule-1 (ICAM-1), vascular cell adhesion molecule-1 (VCAM-1) and E-selectin, further promoting migration; F = ECM protein receptor αvβ3 integrin is upregulated after exposure to growth factors; G = angiostatin, endostatin and antibodies to αvβ3 integrin inhibit endothelial cell proliferation.

creased angiogenesis was noted with the introduction of wild-type p53, which reverted tumors to a dormant phenotype [8]. In the setting of hematological malignancies, the leukemia and/or lymphoma clone may either be destroyed by immune surveillance mechanisms, or develop an angiogenic phenotype (so-called angiogenic 'switch') which favors its survival [9]. The 'switch' may be mediated by the overexpression of angiogenic factors, recruitment of host cells to produce angiogenic factors (e.g. macrophages), and/or mobilization of angiogenic proteins from the extracellular matrix (ECM).

Neovascularization ensues if the balance of proangiogenic factors overcomes the negative effects of the endogenous inhibitors of angiogenesis [2]. The sequence of events is illustrated in figure 1 [10, 11]. During the activation phase of the angiogenic cascade, an endothelial cell lining the wall of an existing small blood vessel is stimulated by a mitogen such as VEGF [12]. Activated endothelial cells then secrete matrix metalloproteinase (MMP) enzymes (e.g. MMP-2 or gelatinase A, and MMP-9 or gelatinase B) which play a significant role in the dissolution of the basement membrane, allowing invasion and migration [13]. VEGF also induces the expression of urokinase-type plasminogen activator and its receptor, promoting further degradation of the ECM.

Proliferation and migration of the endothelial cells result in tube formation; these actions are repeated until a network of tumor-associated capillaries is formed. The resolution phase of angiogenesis involves the maturation and stabilization of the newly formed microvasculature by incorporation of pericytes, formation of junctional complexes between endothelial cells, and reconstitution of the basement membrane. The formation and expansion of the vascular wall is additionally controlled by tie-1 and tie-2 (endothelial cell-specific) receptors, which bind angiopoietin-1 and angiopoietin-2, respectively [14]. Angiopoietin-1 is responsible for the maintenance of established mature vessels, whereas angiopoietin-2 appears to promote new capillary formation after its upregulation is induced by hypoxia or VEGF [14, 15]. Unlike physiological vascularization, malignancy-associated angiogenesis characteristically results in vasculature arranged in tortuous and irregular patterns with blind ends; arteriovenous shunts are not uncommon. These features stem from the enhanced endothelial cell proliferation, decreased number of periendothelial support cells, and increased membrane permeability [2].

Endothelial cells can proliferate rapidly (within several days) during the neovascularization process. The tightly regulated physiological events of embryogenesis [16], placentation, ovulation, and wound healing [17] are associated with increased turnover of endothelial cells. Of the known mitogens, VEGF is considered the most potent endothelial cell activator. Its expression is induced by

Table 1. Endogenous stimulators and inhibitors of angiogenesis

Category	Stimulators	Inhibitors
Cytokines	IL-6, IL-8	IL-1, IL-4, IL-10, IL-12 IFN-α, IFN-β, IFN-γ
Endogenous modulators	αvβ3 integrin Angiopoietin-1 Angiostatin II (AT1 receptor) Endothelin Erythropoietin Hypoxia Nitric oxide synthase Platelet activating factor Prostaglandin E Thrombopoietin	Angiopoietin-2 Angiotensin Angiotensin II (AT2 receptor) Caveolin-1, -2 Endostatin IFN-α Isoflavones Platelet factor-4 Prolactin (16 kD fragment) Thrombospondin Troponin-1
Growth factors	Angiogenin Angiotropin EGF FGF G-CSF HGF PDGF TNF-α VEGF	
Oncogenes	c-*myc*, *ras*, c-*src*, v-*raf*, c-*jun*	*p53*, *Rb*
Proteases, protease inhibitors	Cathepsin Gelatinase A, B Stromelysin Urokinase-type plasminogen activator	TIMP-1, TIMP-2, TIMP-3 Plasminogen activator inhibitor-1
Signal transduction enzymes	Thymidine phosphorylase Farnesyl transferase Geranylgeranyl transferase	
Trace elements	Copper	Zinc

stress signals such as tissue hypoxia, and its fundamental role in physiological processes such as wound healing and embryogenesis is paramount [18]. The loss of only a single VEGF allele leads to embryonic lethality, indicating that this factor plays a critical role in the development of the fetal vascular system [19]. The VEGF family is currently composed of six members. The gene for human VEGF has been localized to chromosome 6p21.3, and contains 8 exons and 7 introns [20, 21]. Alternative splicing produces VEGF isoforms containing 121, 145, 165, 189, or 206 amino acid residues. Isoforms $VEGF_{121}$ and $VEGF_{165}$ have little or no heparin-binding activity, and are secreted by tumor cells [22].

Table 1 lists several other proangiogenic proteins including acidic and basic fibroblast growth factors (aFGF, bFGF), transforming growth factors alpha and beta (TGF-α, TGF-β), angiogenin, epidermal growth factor (EGF), scatter factor/hepatocyte growth factor (HGF), placenta-derived growth factor, interleukin 8 (IL-8), and tumor necrosis factor alpha (TNF-α) [23]. Transcription of VEGF mRNA is induced by several of these cytokines, including platelet-derived growth factor (PDGF), TNF-α, TGF-β and IL-1β. Naturally occurring endogenous inhibitors of angiogenesis include angiostatin, endostatin, interferon alpha (IFN-α), platelet factor 4, thrombospondin, 16-kD fragment of prolactin, and tissue inhibitors of metalloproteinases (TIMP-1, TIMP-2 and TIMP-3).

As anticancer therapy, antiangiogenic agents have been shown to induce tumor regression and prevent the growth of micrometastases [24–27]. Apoptosis of tumor cells in close proximity to endothelium has been demonstrated after therapy with angiogenesis inhibitors targeting the vasculature [28]. These observations underscore the critical role of angiogenesis in promoting tumor proliferation, and the rationale for development of novel therapeutic strategies directed at angiogenesis and tumor-associated vasculature.

Rationale for Antiangiogenic Strategies in Leukemias

The degree of tumor vascularization is an independent prognostic factor for survival in solid tumors such as carcinomas of the breast [29, 30], lung [31], prostate [32, 33] and esophagus [34]. The tumor vascular density also correlates with increased metastases, recurrences, or worse prognosis for carcinomas of the bladder [35, 36], colon [37], and stomach [38], and for melanoma [39]. For leukemias and other hematological malignancies, the pathological correlate of solid tumor vascularization is bone marrow microvessel density (MVD), assessed by staining and quantitating vascular endothelial cells. Methods include staining with hematoxylin and eosin or with the immunostains CD31, CD34, *Ulex europeus* (UEA-1) or factor VIII-related antigen (FVIIIrAg) [40]. Analysis of 'hot spots' (areas with the highest MVD) is usually performed by visual count or computerized image analysis, or both. CD31 not only stains endothelial cells, but also platelets, megakaryocytes and some plasma cells [41]. The CD31 immunostain requires pretreatment with trypsin, potentially resulting in falsely lower readings with this technique. Falsely elevated measurements of vascularity may be obtained by immunostaining immature myeloid cells with CD34, erythroid and stroma cells with UEA-1, and nonspecific staining with polyclonal FVIIIrAg [10, 42].

Bearing in mind the caveats regarding interpretation of the results obtained with the various techniques and use of proper controls, increased marrow vascularity has been reported in various leukemias and myeloproliferative disorders, and appears to be independent of marrow cellularity [43, 44]. Perez-Atayde et al. [43] studied the vascularity (as assessed by FVIIIrAg staining) of bone marrow biopsies obtained from 40 children with newly diagnosed acute lymphocytic leukemia (ALL). Median MVD was 42 counts per field in childhood ALL versus 6 per field in marrows of children with solid tumors or lymphomas not involving the marrow ($p = 0.0001$). The MVD of 'hot spots' (highest vascularity) was also higher in ALL (51 vs. 8; $p = 0.0001$) compared with controls. Computer-aided three-dimensional reconstruction model of marrow vascularity showed complex arborizing branching of microvessels in leukemic samples (vs. single straight microvessels without branching in normal controls). Serial assessments of MVD were limited to a few patients; no significant changes were observed. As another measure of angiogenesis, serial measurements of urinary bFGF were performed. Levels were high prior to chemotherapy in all 22 leukemic patients, were variable during induction, and were decreased at the time of complete remission (CR).

Elevated levels of various proangiogenic factors, including but not limited to VEGF, bFGF and TNF-α have been reported in hematological malignancies in addition to the increased marrow vascularity, and have been correlated with worse survival in some studies (table 2) [43–80]. Mesa et al. [59] demonstrated that increased marrow vascularity in myelofibrosis was associated with increased splenomegaly and shorter survival. Rajkumar et al. [70] showed that increased marrow angiogenesis was associated with shorter survival in patients with newly diagnosed multiple myeloma. Aguayo et al. [51] demonstrated that intracellular levels of VEGF in leukemic blasts of patients with acute myelogenous leukemia (AML) were higher than mononuclear cells from controls. There was no correlation between increased VEGF levels and established prognostic factors. Elevated levels greater than 2.5 pg/ml and increasing levels of VEGF were independently associated with worse survival by multivariate analysis. Table 2 details the correlation of increased angiogenic factors with worse progression-free or overall survival observed in myelodysplastic syndrome (MDS) [52, 53], chronic myelogenous leukemia (CML) [56–58], chronic lymphocytic leukemia (CLL) [63], multiple myeloma [69, 70], and non-Hodgkin's lymphoma [75–77].

However, these angiogenic factors can be produced by normal hematological cells such as monocytes, T cells, neutrophils, platelets and megakaryocytes [81]. In fact, to what extent the increased levels of angiogenic factors is physiological in hematological disorders is not known [82, 83]. bFGF is a hematopoietic cytokine produced by stromal cells, megakaryocytes and cells of the granulocytic lineage. It stimulates stromal cell proliferation, megakaryopoiesis and myelopoiesis in long-term bone marrow cultures [84]. TNF-α, a primary cytokine secreted by activated macrophages, enhances neoangiogenesis by induction of endothelial production and secretion of collagenase, urokinase-type plasminogen activator, and plasminogen activator-inhibitor-1 [85]. This cytokine also induces the expression of bFGF mRNA (and collagenase or IL-6 mRNA) in human omental microvascular cells, and interacts with other proliferative cytokines such as IL-6 [85].

Data in support of pathological angiogenesis in hematological malignancies includes the secretion of hematopoietic growth factors such as GM-CSF or G-CSF and

Table 2. Evidence for increased angiogenesis in leukemias and lymphomas

Disease	Angiogenesis markers	Prognostic associations with survival	Ref. No.
ALL	↑ Marrow MVD	–	43, 44
	↑ Urinary bFGF, angiostatin	–	45
	↑ VEGF, IL-6 secretion by stromal cells	–	46
	↑ TNF-α secretion by leukemia cells	–	46
	↑ Angiogenesis with ALL plasma	–	47
AML	↑ Marrow MVD	–	48–50
	↑ Cellular VEGF	Shorter	51
	↑ VEGFR-1 (relative to MDS)	–	52
	↑ Plasma endostatin	Shorter	53
MDS	↑ Marrow MVD	–	54
	↑ Marrow VEGF	Shorter	52
	↑ VEGFR-2 (compared with AML)	–	52
	↑ Plasma endostatin	Shorter	53
CML	↑ Marrow MVD	–	44, 55
	↑ Marrow VEGF protein	Shorter (in CP only)	56
	↑ Marrow VEGFR-1	Shorter (in AP/BP)	57
	↑ Marrow VEGFR-2	Shorter (in CP only)	57
	↑ Tie-1 protein	Shorter (in CP only)	58
Myelofibrosis	↑ Marrow MVD	Shorter	55, 59
	↑ Serum VEGF	–	60
CLL	↑ Marrow MVD	–	61
	↑ Cellular VEGF	Longer	62
	↑ Serum VEGF	Shorter progression-free	63
	↑ mRNA VEGF	–	64
	↑ Cellular and plasma bFGF	–	65
Hairy cell leukemia	↑ Marrow mononuclear TGF-β	–	66
	↑ Marrow and serum bFGF	–	67
Multiple myeloma	↑ Marrow MVD	Shorter progression-free	68–71
	↑ MMP-2 secretion	Shorter progression-free	72
	↑ Marrow VEGF	–	73
Non-Hodgin's lymphoma	↑ MVD	–	74
	↑ Serum VEGF	Shorter	75,76
	↑ Serum bFGF	Shorter	77

AP = Accelerated phase; BP = blastic phase; CP = chronic phase.

angiogenic factors such as VEGF and VEGF-C by AML leukemia blasts in vitro [83]. Bellamy et al. [86] demonstrated the expression of mRNA and protein for VEGF in 12 hematopoietic tumor cell lines including ALL (HUT 78, Jurkat, Molt4, CCRF-CEM, NALM 16), Burkitt's lymphoma (Raji, Ramos), histiocytic lymphoma (U937), promyelocytic leukemia (HL-60), CML (K562), and plasma cell dyscrasias (8226, ARH77). The expression of bFGF was detected in HUT 78, Ramos, U937, HL-60, K562, 8226 and ARH77. Vacca et al. [87] confirmed the angiogenic potential of human lymphoproliferative cell lines (Namalwa, Raji, Daudi, LIK, SB, CEM, Jurkat, U266), particularly with the expression of MMP-2 and/or MMP-9. Both bFGF and VEGF were secreted by Raji, LIK, SB, CEM and Jurkat cells. Daudi and U266 only produced bFGF, whereas Namalwa cells produced VEGF alone.

Table 3. Marrow vascularity and relative (compared with controls) plasma[1] levels of angiogenic factors

Disease	Vascularity	VEGF	bFGF	HGF	TNF-α
ALL	+	–	–	++	++
AML	+	–	–	++	–
CLL	–	+	+++	++	+++
CML	+++	+++	+	++	++
Chronic myelomonocytic leukemia	++	++	–	+++	+
MDS	++	–	–	++	–
Myelofibrosis	+++	+++	–	++	+++

– = Similar to controls; + = mildly elevated; ++ = moderately elevated, +++ = markedly elevated.

[1] Release of VEGF from platelets during coagulation may affect serum levels.

Receptors for VEGF (VEGFR) are primarily found on endothelial cells; however, hematopoietic stem cells, megakaryocytes, platelets and monocytes also harbor VEGFRs [82]. There are at least two tyrosine kinase receptors with affinity for VEGF that undergo autophosphorylation upon binding, VEGFR-1 (FLT-1) and VEGFR-2 (FLK/KDR). The biologic activities of endothelial cells appear to be mediated by VEGFR-2 [88]. Recent reports have identified VEGFRs on malignant cells of ovarian tumors and leukemia blasts (FLT-1), and bFGF receptors on human leukemia cells [89–91]. The presence of VEGFRs and bFGFRs on leukemia blasts suggests the possibility of an autocrine pathway by which malignant cells may stimulate their own growth.

There is significant heterogeneity in levels of soluble mediators and marrow vascularity among the various leukemias (table 3). Pruneri et al. [54] reported that the intermediate vascularity of bone marrows from patients with MDS compared with increased vascularity in AML suggests a correlation between angiogenesis and progression of disease; however, other investigators detected no difference in vascularity between MDS samples and controls. Aguayo et al. [44] observed that in CLL, the marrow vascularity was similar to controls despite increased levels of angiogenic factors. In contrast, Kini et al. [61] reported increased marrow vascularity in their CLL bone marrow cases. Technical differences could account for the discrepancy in results observed by different investigators.

Although several investigators have demonstrated that increased levels of angiogenic factors or marrow vascularity are associated with worse outcome, few have been able to correlate these findings with other biologic features of the leukemia, such as abnormal karyotype, immunophenotype and/or oncogene expression. In CLL, bFGF has been shown to upregulate the expression of the antiapoptotic protein bcl-2, resulting in increased leukemia cell survival [92]. Elevated intracellular levels of bFGF have correlated clinically with advanced stage and resistance to fludarabine [93]. Munshi et al. [94] correlated increased angiogenesis with trisomy 13, β_2-microglobulin, and C-reactive protein. Mangi and Newland [10] reported a correlation between marrow angiogenesis and extramedullary disease in chronic myelomonocytic leukemia. These studies, and others, further support the hypothesis that targeting angiogenesis may be a therapeutic intervention which improves outcome.

Role of Bone Marrow Stroma and Endothelial Cells

The normal vascular bed in the bone marrow forms a sinusoidal network supporting the hematopoietic cells [95–97]. Endothelial cells and hematopoietic cells have a common cell origin in embryogenesis (so-called hemangioblast) [98]. Bone marrow-derived endothelial cell progenitors may participate in both physiological and pathological neovascularization. The formation of vascular structures and the close contact of hematopoietic foci have been described in long-term bone marrow cultures [99, 100]. Mice deficient in FLF-1/KDR VEGFRs manifest failure of blood-island formation in addition to angiogenesis [101].

Normal hematopoietic progenitors interact with stromal cells, which then produce bFGF and cytokines, including IL-6, IL-8 and others [102]. Angiogenic factors of the FGF-type induce mesoderm and stimulate the formation

Table 4. Antiangiogenic agents: direct endothelial cell, cytokine and tyrosine kinase effects

Agent	Other mechanism(s) of action	Comment(s)
Direct inhibitors of endothelial cells		
Angiostatin	Induction of apoptosis of endothelial cells and tumor cells Inhibition of endothelial cell migration and tubule formation Inhibition of matrix-enhanced plasminogen activation	38-kD fragment plasminogen
Combretastatin	Induction of apoptosis in proliferating cells	
Endostatin	Inhibition of endothelial cells	20-kD fragment type XVIII collagen
FTI		
L-778, 123	Blocks endothelial cell migration/proliferation	Phase I trials in refractory leukemias
SCH66336		Phase I trial in MDS, CMML
R11577		Phase II trials in MDS, CMML, CML, multiple myeloma, angiogenic myeloid metaplasia
Penicillamine	Urokinase inhibitor; sulfhydryl groups bind copper Blocks endothelial cell migration/proliferation Inhibits uPA	
Squalamine	Inhibition of sodium-hydrogen pump, NHE3	Extract from dogfish shark liver
Thalidomide	Inhibition of VEGF, bFGF, TNF-α Stimulation of IFN-γ and IL-2	Activity in multiple myeloma, myelodysplasia
TNP-470	Synthetic analogue fumagillin Inhibition of endothelial cell growth	In vitro cytotoxicity human leukemia cell lines
Block activators of angiogenesis		
Angiozyme	Attenuation of mRNA of VEGF receptors	
Anti-VEGF	Monoclonal antibody to VEGF	Recognizes all isoforms VEGF Phase II MDS, CML-BP
IM862	Inhibition of bFGF and VEGF production Upregulation of IL-12	
IFN-α	Inhibition of bFGF and VEGF production	
PTK787/ZK22584	Blocks VEGFR signaling	
SU5416	Blocks VEGFR (flk-1/KDR) signaling	Phase II hematological malignancies
SU6668	Blocks VEGF, FGF and PDGFR signaling	Phase I advanced malignancies; oral
Inhibitors endothelial-specific integrin/survival signaling		
ABT-627	Endothelin receptor antagonist	
EMD121974	Small molecule blocker of αvβ3 integrin	
Vitaxin	Antibody to αvβ3 integrin Induction endothelial cell apoptosis	
Miscellaneous		
IL-12	Upregulation IFN-γ; inhibition production of MMP	
PNU-145156E	Blocks angiogenesis induced by Tat protein	

FTI = Farnesyl transferase inhibitor; CMML = chronic myelomonocytic leukemia; uPA = urokinase-type plasminogen activator; CML-BP = chronic myelogenous leukemia in blast phase.

of blood cells. bFGF is a potent mitogen for stromal cells and significantly delays their senescence. In addition, bFGF enhances the effects of IL-3 and GM-CSF on normal myeloid precursors via FGF receptors, stimulating granulopoiesis and megakaryopoiesis [21]. Of interest, the gene for acidic FGF is located on the long arm of chromosome 5, which is deleted in the 5q– syndrome subtype of MDS, typically characterized by megakaryopoiesis rather than thrombocytopenia [103]. Macrophages also play a role in tumor angiogenesis by the secretion of proteases, growth

Table 5. Antiangiogenic agents: MMP inhbitors

Agent	Clinical trial(s)	Comments
AG 3340	Combination with chemotherapy in NSCLC, prostate	Synthetic
Bay 12-9566	NSCLC; small cell lung, pancreatic, ovarian carcinomas	Synthetic MMP-2 and MMP-9 inhibitor
BMS-275291	Phase II/III NSCLC, phase I refractory leukemias	Synthetic
COL-3	Phase I/II gliomas	Synthetic; Tetracycline® derivative
Marimastat (BB-2516)	Phase III small cell lung and breast carcinoma	Synthetic; blocks TNF-α convertase
MM1270		Synthetic
Neovastat (AE941)	Phase III renal cell carcinoma, phase III NSCLC	Natural, shark cartilage extract

NSCLC = Non-small cell lung carcinoma.

factors (e.g., TNF-α, PDGF), and other cytokines. PDGF stimulates the proliferation of bone marrow fibroblasts, a pathological process identified in agnogenic myeloid metaplasia and other myelofibrotic states [21].

Leukemia-specific angiogenesis may depend upon an interaction between marrow stromal cells and the leukemia cells, which impart a survival advantage to the latter. Endothelial cells and osteoblasts in the marrow stroma exposed to VEGF increase mRNA expression of GM-CSF, G-CSF, IL-6, IL-8 and/or stem cell factor (SCF; ligand for c-kit) [104]. These cytokines, in turn, can stimulate the proliferation of myeloid and lymphoid malignant cells. Endothelial cells express peroxisome-proliferator-activated receptor-gamma (PPAR-γ), a nuclear receptor involved in the transcriptional activation of differentiation-associated genes. Natural PPAR-γ ligands, such as prostaglandin J2, activate PPAR-γ and inhibit endothelial cell proliferation as well as new capillary formation in the bone marrow stroma derived from patients with ALL [105]. Thus, pharmacologic agents which activate PPAR-γ could disrupt the stromal endothelial-leukemia cell interactions which lead to angiogenesis and proliferation. When in direct contact with the leukemia clone, endothelial cells also appear to prevent apoptosis, by increasing the ratio of antiapoptotic genes (e.g., *bcl-2* and *bcl-x*) to proapoptotic genes (e.g., *bax* and *bad*) [106].

Angiogenic modulators in the plasma isolated from ALL-involved marrow aspirates, supernatants from ALL cell cultures and supernatants from ALL bone marrow stroma all induced proliferation of vascular endothelial cells and marrow endothelial cells in vitro [47]. Primary ALL cells expressed mRNA for VEGF, TGF-α, angiopoietin-1 and angiopoietin 2 (but not bFGF or aFGF). Leukemic bone marrow stromal cells expressed mRNA for all the angiogenic modulators studied, including bFGF and aFGF. ALL leukemia cells cultured in the absence of marrow endothelium cells did not survive, stressing the importance of stromal interactions for continued proliferation of the malignant clone.

Antiangiogenic Strategies in Hematological Malignancies

Several steps of the angiogenic cascade can be modulated (fig. 1). Although some molecules were designed with a specific function (e.g., SU5416 which inhibits the FLK-1 VEGFR), others have additional mechanisms of action besides their purported antiangiogenic properties (e.g., thalidomide, discussed below). Agents that inhibit the proliferation or response of normal endothelial cells to stimuli include those that target endoglin, integrins and VEGFR complexes (table 4). Strategies include blockade of growth factor-mediated angiogenesis by inhibiting VEGFR signaling pathways, neutralizing VEGF (monoclonal antibodies or dominant negative receptors), or inhibiting bFGF. Direct administration of (or transfer of DNA that encodes for) endogenous inhibitors (e.g., angiostatin), synthetic inhibitors of endothelial cell division (e.g., derivatives of fumagillin such as TNP-470), or inhibitors of endothelial cell-mediated ECM breakdown (e.g., MMP inhibitors) could block angiogenesis (table 4, 5).

Endothelial cell-specific receptor tyrosine kinases and their ligands play a critical role in angiogenesis, and are expressed at high levels in tumor blood vessels. All of these molecules have an extracellular ligand-binding domain, a transmembrane domain, and an intracellular tyrosine kinase domain. Upon ligand binding, the receptors dimerize, the tyrosine kinase is activated, and the receptors become autophoshorylated. The activity of the specific receptor tyrosine kinase leads to subsequent cellular events such as proliferation, differentiation and/or morphogenesis. The VEGF tyrosine kinase receptors FLT-1 (VEGFR-1) and KDR/FLK-1 (VEGFR-2) are expressed in endothelial cells of blood vessels, and both are required for normal development of embryonic vasculature. FLT-4 (VEGFR-3), previously postulated to be restricted to lymphatic endothelium, has been detected on AML blasts, and binds VEGF-C and VEGF-D [107].

Human uterine smooth muscle cells and retinal pigment cells express both FLT-1 and KDR [108, 109]. FLK-1 receptors which lack the intracellular kinase domain block the activation of endogenous FLK-1 receptor activity in cultured cells, inhibiting the growth of tumors implanted subcutaneously in nude mice [110]. Any tumors that formed had significantly reduced vessel density. Tie receptor kinases have also been reported to play a role in both hematopoiesis and angiogenesis, particularly in myeloid human leukemia cell lines [111]. Tie expression has been detected in primitive human hematopoietic progenitor cells [112, 113]. Enhanced expression of Tie receptors Tie-1 and Tie-2/Tek has been demonstrated in tumor vasculature, and may be a potential therapeutic target [114].

Apoptosis of those endothelial cells directly contributing to active tumor angiogenesis induces 100-fold tumor cell death [114]. Thus, directly targeting the unique vasculature of malignant clones may be of therapeutic benefit. In addition, this strategy may bypass the acquired cytotoxic drug resistance typically observed with chemotherapy. Phage display libraries can identify unique peptide sequences specific to tumor-associated vasculature, allowing administration of targeted therapy (e.g, guided chemotherapy or immunotoxin delivery) [115]. Saiki et al. [116] reported that peptides containing the integrin recognition sequence Arg-Gly-Asp (RGD) can inhibit tumor angiogenesis. The $\alpha v\beta 3$ and $\alpha v\beta 5$ integrins are upregulated in angiogenic tumor endothelial cells, and inhibition of αv integrins by antibodies, cyclic RGD peptides, or RGD peptidomimetics can block neovascularization [117, 118].

Strategies combining angiogenesis inhibitors with cytotoxic chemotherapy, biologic agents, or other antiangiogenic agents exploit (1) different cellular targets, (2) lack of cross-resistance, (3) lack of additive myelosuppression enabling full dose administration of the agents, and (4) possible synergy or additive effects. Clinical trials employing these tactics are underway in hematological malignancies.

Development, Interpretation and Monitoring of Clinical Trials of Antiangiogenic Agents in Leukemia

Angiogenesis inhibitors differ from conventional cytotoxic chemotherapy agents, and require evaluation in clinical trials with an approach such as 'cytostatic paradigm'. Traditionally, objective response has been the surrogate for clinical activity. In clinical trials with antiangiogenic agents, however, time to disease progression and overall survival are more appropriate endpoint(s) (table 6). Determining improvements in time to progression, however, can be problematic owing to the heterogeneity of the historical database, and the inherent bias in intensity and frequency of disease assessments. Frequently, modulators of angiogenesis require prolonged administration to demonstrate clinical activity, thus potentially limiting the benefit in rapidly proliferative diseases.

Interpretation of antiangiogenic endpoints such as changes in VEGF levels or marrow vascular density requires knowledge of other pathophysiological processes influencing these measurements. For example, higher VEGF concentrations are observed in serum compared with plasma samples owing to the release of VEGF from platelets during activation of the coagulation cascade [119]. Longitudinal analysis of various angiogenic factors and marrow vascularity can be influenced by disease type, therapy administered, timing of collections, and method of detection [120].

Some antiangiogenic agents may not be able to induce tumor regression, but may induce tumor dormancy or stabilization. Therefore, a toxicity profile favoring prolonged administration is paramount. Monitoring for potential toxicities related to antiangiogenic agents in general should include changes in menstruation and fertility in women of child-bearing potential, worsening peripheral vascular disease (e.g., diabetes mellitus), impaired wound healing, or blunted neovascularization following acute myocardial infarction. Thromboembolic events such as pulmonary embolus and deep venous thrombosis have been reported with antiangiogenic agents, including thalidomide; however, the majority of cases were associated with known risk factors such as the presence of antiphospholipid/anticardiolipin antibodies or trauma [121]. In vivo animal models have demonstrated that resolution of venous thrombi is associated with ingrowth of capillaries, in addition to elevated VEGF and bFGF levels [122]. Thus, angiogenic inhibitors could inhibit this physiological process of recanalization and promote venous thrombosis. Further studies are needed to delineate the associa-

Table 6. Comparison of cytotoxic chemotherapy with angiogenesis inhibitors

Parameter	Chemotherapy	Angiogenesis inhibitors
Onset of effect	Rapid	Slower
Target	Tumor cells	Endothelial cell receptors
Mechanism(s) of action	Specific to agent	Multiple Direct inhibition endothelial cell Modulation of αvβ3 integrin Inhibition MMP Inhibition bFGF, VEGF and/or TNF-α Neutralization of VEGF or VEGFR
Drug resistance	Commonly acquired	Less likely due to multiple targets without cross resistance
Tumor milieu		
Hypoxia Cell kinetics Tumor cell burden	All critical factors in efficacy	Hypoxia and cell kinetics not important Tumor cell burden may be factor
Toxicity		
Alopecia	Frequent	Rare
Gastrointestinal	Mucositis, nausea, diarrhea	Agent specific
Myelosuppression	Frequent	Rare
Wound healing	Delayed	Delayed
Clinical trial endpoint		
Phase I	Maximum tolerated dose	Maximum biologic effect
Phase II	Tumor reduction	Time to progression and survival
Combination	Overlapping toxicities, reduced doses required for drug combinations	Synergy with chemotherapy, radiation therapy, other antiangiogenesis agents

tion. The use of low dose prophylactic anticoagulation (e.g., warfarin 1 mg orally daily or low molecular weight heparin subcutaneously) has been advocated by some investigators in the absence of contraindications (e.g., thrombopenia related to underlying leukemia), particularly with antiangiogenic agents requiring a central venous catheter for administration.

Antiangiogenesis Agents under Study in Hematological Malignancies

Chemotherapeutic Agents with Antiangiogenic Activity

Assessments of the degree of residual angiogenesis after chemotherapy for hematological malignancies have not consistently correlated with outcome. Reduction in marrow MVD was not observed with induction chemotherapy in childhood ALL [43] (although reductions in bFGF were observed in those who achieved CR), or with autologous transplantation in multiple myeloma [68]. In contrast, Padró et al. [48] reported normalization (even after 16 days) of marrow vascularity after induction chemotherapy for newly diagnosed AML.

Various traditional chemotherapy compounds used to treat leukemias have putative antiangiogenic activity (table 7). In vivo methods such as chick chorioallantoic membrane assays, corneal micropocket assays, matrix implant assays, and tumor xenograft models allow identification of drugs which inhibit VEGF- or bFGF-induced angiogenesis [123–125]. However, for a chemotherapeutic agent to be considered antiangiogenic, its antiproliferative or other effects on endothelial cells should be achieved prior to cytotoxic effects on the malignant cells. Agents which demonstrate cytotoxic effects at lower doses but do not exert antiangiogenic effects until significant dose escalation should not be considered antiangiogenic.

Table 7 illustrates a partial list of chemotherapy agents used in hematological malignancies and their potential mechanisms of action related to angiogenesis [126–132]. Several drugs demonstrating cytotoxicity to tumor cells when administered intermittently at higher doses are antiangiogenic when administered at low doses over pro-

Table 7. Antiangiogenic effects of chemotherapy agents used in leukemias

Agent	Antiangiogenic mechanisms	Leukemia(s)	Ref. No.
Topotecan	Inhibits EC proliferation at low concentrations	AML, MDS	126
Doxorubicin	Increases EC nitric oxide (enhanced superoxide) Decreases collagen synthesis Inhibits MMP-1	ALL, NHL	127, 128
Methotrexate	Inhibits EC proliferation	ALL	129
6-Mercaptopurine	Inhibits EC proliferation Alters FGF-2-induced intracellular signaling	ALL	130
Vincristine	Decreases MMP-2 and MMP-9 secretion	ALL, NHL	131
Cyclophosphamide	Inhibits EC proliferation Increases VEGF, CD31 expression	ALL, NHL	132

EC = Endothelial cell; NHL = non-Hodgkin's lymphoma.

longed exposure periods. For example, an alternative antiangiogenic schedule has been described for cyclophosphamide. An in vivo animal model of drug-resistant leukemia demonstrated eradication of the established malignancy 3-fold more effectively with the administration of the 'antiangiogenic schedule' compared with the conventional maximum tolerated dose [133]. In this study, it was hypothesized that resistance mechanisms were bypassed due to the sequential induction of apoptosis of first the tumor-associated endothelial cells, followed by death of the tumor cells.

IFN-α and IL-12

Fidler et al. [134, 135] demonstrated the antiangiogenic activity of IFN-α in addition to its antiproliferative potential; the biologic effect of angiosuppression was best achieved with prolonged administration at low rather than high doses. In hairy cell leukemia, the efficacy of low-dose chronic IFN-α administration has been well established [136]. Di Raimondo et al. [137] demonstrated lower values of VEGF and HGF in patients with CML treated with IFN-α therapy when compared with those receiving alternative agents such as hydroxyurea. In CML IFN-α induced restoration of β_1 integrin-mediated adhesion of leukemia progenitors to the stroma, indicating the importance of stromal interactions in suppressing the leukemia [138].

IL-12 (Genetics Institute, Cambridge, Mass., USA) is a multifunctional cytokine produced by macrophages and B lymphocytes. IL-12 stimulates proliferation of T lymphocytes and natural killer cells, IFN-γ production, and cytolytic lymphocyte (Th1-type helper) response [139]. It has been reported to inhibit angiogenesis in an in vivo mouse model of corneal neovascularization induced by bFGF [140]. IL-12 targets the tumor vasculature via IFN-γ and downstream cytokines such as IFN-inducible protein-10 [139]. Combinations of IL-12 with other angiogenesis inhibitors (e.g., vasostatin) produced tumor responses in athymic mice [141]. Clinical trials of IL-12 in refractory CML are underway.

Thalidomide

In 1994, the antiangiogenic potential of thalidomide was discovered when D'Amato et al. [142] demonstrated that thalidomide (Celgene, Warren, N.J., USA) inhibited bFGF-induced angiogenesis in a rabbit cornea micropocket assay. Later, investigators reported that it also inhibited VEGF in a murine model of corneal vascularization [143]. Thalidomide inhibits TNF-α production by stimulated monocytes, macrophages and neutrophils by (1) accelerated degradation of TNF-α mRNA, (2) binding to α_1-acid glycoproteins with intrinsic anti-TNF-α activity, and (3) decreased binding activity of NFκB which controls the activation of the TNF-α gene [144–146].

Thalidomide was explored in other hematological disorders after Singhal et al. [147] demonstrated significant activity of single agent oral thalidomide in relapsed or refractory multiple myeloma and plasma cell leukemias [148]. Preliminary activity in pilot studies of thalidomide in relapsed or refractory AML or MDS was observed [149]. Subsequently, a randomized trial of liposomal daunorubicin (DaunoXome, Gilead, Calif.) and ara-C induction chemotherapy with or without thalidomide (400 mg daily escalated to 600 mg as tolerated) was conducted in poor risk [abnormal karyotype other than t(15;17), t(8;21) or inversion 16] patients with newly diagnosed AML

[150]. No significant difference in CR rate (44 vs. 53%, respectively) was observed either with or without thalidomide.

Preliminary activity of single agent thalidomide has been reported in myeloproliferative disorders, myelofibrosis and Waldenström's macroglobulinemia [151]. Particularly encouraging results have been observed with the use of thalidomide in early-stage MDS. Raza et al. [152] reported preliminary results in 61 patients with MDS treated with 100 to 400 mg of thalidomide daily. Seventeen of 25 evaluable patients (68%) responded with improvements in at least one cell lineage. Transfusion independence was reported. Some responses were not manifest until 3 months of therapy. Responders had lower pretreatment marrow apoptosis and lower serum levels of TGF-β and TNF-α compared with nonresponders [153]. Additional confirmatory phase II and III trials with single agent thalidomide in MDS are being conducted. Combination strategies for such patients are being explored, including thalidomide given with other biologic agents (e.g., Enbrel) or chemotherapeutics (e.g., topotecan).

Owing to the multiple actions of thalidomide, it is difficult to determine which mechanism is responsible for its activity. Thalidomide analogues designed for increased efficacy and decreased toxicity (e.g. lack of teratogenicity and decreased sedation) are currently in development [151]. The first class of compounds are immunomodulating drugs (ImiDs™) such as CDC 501, which inhibit TNF-α with a 10,000-fold increased potency compared with the parent compound. ImiDs™ resemble thalidomide in their ability to inhibit IL-1β, IL-6, and IL-12 and enhance IL-10, IL-2, and IFN-γ. Costimulation of T cells is significantly enhanced compared with thalidomide. The second group of thalidomide-related TNF-α inhibitors are the selective cytokine inhibitory drugs (SelCIDs™). These agents (such as CDC 801) inhibit phosphodiesterase-4, an enzyme which influences the overproduction of TNF-α. These agents are currently entering phase II trials in Crohn's disease (CDC 801), MDS (CDC 801) and multiple myeloma (CDC 501).

SU5416 and SU6668

SU5416 and SU6668 (Sugen, South San Francisco, Calif., USA) are potent small molecule inhibitors of receptor tyrosine kinases that play a role in intracellular signal transduction. SU5416 inactivates VEGFR-2 receptor flk-1/KDR by binding to the adenine binding site of the intracellular catalytic core [153, 154]. SU6668 is an oral inhibitor with a broader spectrum of activity against VEGFR-1, VEGFR-2 and PDGFR. In vitro, SU5416 and SU6668 inhibited autophosphorylation of the SCF receptor c-kit in MO7E cells/AML blasts and SCF-induced proliferation of MO7E cells [155, 156]. Apoptosis [measured by appearance of activated caspase-3 and cleavage of poly-(ADP-ribose) polymerase] of SCF-treated MO7E cells/AML blasts occurred in a dose-dependent manner.

Phase I data included that from over 60 patients treated with SU5416 at doses ranging from 4.4 to 190 mg/m^2, nearly all with twice weekly administration [157]. Dose-limiting toxicities at the highest dose included symptoms such as projectile vomiting, severe headache and nausea which were unresponsive to standard interventions. These events occurred within 3–6 h following the first dose, and resolved within 24–48 h. Severe myelosuppression was rarely observed (grade 3–4 anemia 2%, leukopenia 1.5%, thrombocytopenia 2.2%). Hypersensitivity events were related to the excipients of the formulation (polyoxyethylated castor oil, Cremophor 7); all patients were premedicated with antihistamines (H1 and H2 antagonists) and dexamethasone prior to each infusion.

Fiedler et al. [158] reported a phase II study of SU5416 in 14 patients with AML given 145 mg/m^2 twice weekly for 4 weeks. In general, the treatment was well tolerated except for bone pain (n = 3), grade 4 pancreatitis (n = 1), or grade 4 hepatotoxicity (n = 1). Five patients (36%) had a partial response (>50% decrease in peripheral and marrow blasts), 3 (21%) were nonresponders after 4 weeks of therapy, and 6 (43%) progressed on therapy. Phase II clinical trials of SU5416 and SU6668 are underway in patients with refractory acute leukemias and MDS, Philadelphia-chromosome negative myeloproliferative disorders, CML in blast transformation, agnogenic myeloid metaplasia and multiple myeloma.

Anti-VEGF Monoclonal Antibody

Bevacizumab (rhuMab VEGF, Genentech, San Francisco, Calif., USA) is a recombinant glycosylated humanized anti-VEGF IgG1 monoclonal antibody. The antigen-binding complementarity determining regions from a murine monoclonal antibody recognizes all VEGF isoforms. Bevacizumab has a high affinity for VEGF, but fails to recognize FGF, EGF, HGF or PDGF. The agent has a long half-life without evidence of immunogenicity. A phase I dose escalation study was conducted in 25 patients with 90-min infusions days 0, 28, 35 and 42 [159]. Dose-limiting toxicities were not observed in weekly doses up to 10 mg/kg. Toxicities observed included mild headache, fatigue, nausea and low-grade fever. Three tumor-related hemorrhagic episodes were observed. One responder with renal cell carcinoma had a 33% reduction in tumor size. Combination studies with chemotherapy agents are ongoing in solid tumors. In hematological malignancies, phase II studies of Bevacizumab in MDS and myeloid blast phase of CML (the latter in combination with idarubicin and ara-C) are ongoing.

COX Inhibitors

COX-1 and COX-2 are enzymes putatively involved in the angiogenesis process [160]. COX-2 mediates the conversion of arachidonic acid into prostaglandin G_2, which is subsequently converted to prostaglandin H_2, then thromboxane A_2. In vitro, COX-2 was shown to stimulate colon cancer cells to release angiogenic prostaglandins, which induce migration and tube formation of endothelial cells. Inhibitors of COX-1 and COX-2 such as nonsteroidal anti-inflammatory drugs blocked this effect; however, additional prostaglandin-independent effects on angiogenesis by COX-2 were suspected, since only partial reversal of the inhibition was achieved with reexposure to prostaglandins [161]. Increased COX-2 levels have been observed in various malignancies, suggesting that inhibitors may be of therapeutic benefit [162].

TNP-470

TNP-470 is a derivative of fumagillin, a naturally occurring substance which inhibits endothelial cell growth [163]. Inhibition of bFGF- and PDGF-stimulated endothelial proliferation has been demonstrated. Toxicities observed in the phase I studies included fatigue and dose-related CNS effects (dizziness, imbalance, ataxia and encephalopathy) [164]. Phase II trials of TNP-470 have been reported to show efficacy in cervical cancer [165] and Kaposi's sarcoma [166]. In vitro data with TNP-470 has demonstrated moderate cytotoxicity with human leukemia HL-60, HL-60/ADR, HL-60/VCR and myeloma ARH77 cell lines [167], suggesting a possible role in hematological malignancies.

Farnesyl Transferase Inhibitors, Other Miscellaneous Agents

Activation of the *ras* oncogene is an important pathway to stimulate angiogenesis, as the tumorigenicity of the *ras* oncogene may be VEGF-dependent. The anticancer activity of farnesyl tranferase inhibitors appears to stem from their ability to inhibit farnesylation of various proteins that mediate signal transduction, growth, apoptosis and angiogenesis [168]. Dose-dependent suppression of angiogenesis by farnesyl transferase inhibitors has been demonstrated in vitro via direct inhibition of endothelial cell proliferation [169]. Several farnesyl transferase inhibitors are under investigation in clinical trials (table 4).

Arsenicals have resurged as antileukemia agents, particularly in acute promyelocytic leukemia. In vitro, arsenic trioxide (As_2O_3) demonstrated antiangiogenic activity by inhibiting production of VEGF either by direct suppression of human umbilical cells or their interactions with the vasculature and/or stroma [170]. Direct effects of As_2O_3 on tumor vasculature was demonstrated in fibrosarcoma grown in BABL/c mice, where tumor perfusion studies demonstrated vascular shutdown in the tumor at 2 and 6 h, leading to central necrosis of the tumor [171].

Future Directions

Combination of antiangiogenic drugs with different mechanisms of action may lead to synergistic effects [172]. In addition, a combination of anti-angiogenic agents with traditional chemotherapy agents appear more efficacious than the components given as single agents [173]. Enhancement of the effects of targeted therapies may be observed. For example, a VEGF-diphtheria toxin conjugate (VEGF-DT385) inhibited the growth of tumor xenografts in nude mice significantly more than diphtheria toxin alone [174]. Identification of targets on endothelial cells specific to tumor vasculature (e.g., $\alpha_v\beta_3$ integrin, E-selectin, VEGFR) exploit the delivery of specific biologic agents directly to malignant clone, reducing systemic toxicity [114]. Gene therapy has the potential to modulate angiogenesis by transduction of cDNA-encoding antiangiogenic proteins (e.g., endostatin, angiostatin, or PF-4) or antisense VEGF via adenoviral or retroviral vectors [175, 176]. The study of angiogenic markers of progression in hematological malignancies, and the use of angiosuppressive therapy may improve outcome in these entities.

References

1 Folkman J: Tumor angiogenesis: Therapeutic complications. N Engl J Med 1971;285:1182–1186.
2 Folkman J: Angiogenesis in cancer, vascular, rheumatoid, and other disease. Nat Med 1995; 1:27–31.
3 Folkman J: Seminars in Medicine of the Beth Israel Hospital, Boston. Clinical applications of research on angiogenesis. N Engl J Med 1995; 333:1757–1763.
4 Boehm T, Folkman J, Browder T, O'Reilly MS: Antiangiogenic therapy of experimental cancer does not induce acquired drug resistance. Nature 1997;390:404–407.
5 Cheresh DA: Death to a blood vessel, death to a tumor. Nat Med 1998;4:395–396.
6 Benjamin LE, Golijanin D, Itin A, Pode D, Keshet E: Selective ablation of immature blood vessels in established human tumors follows vascular endothelial growth factor withdrawal. J Clin Invest 1999;103:159–165.
7 Grant SW, Kyshtoobayeva AS, Kurosaki T, Jakowatz J, Fruehauf JP: Mutant p53 correlates with reduced expression of thrombospondin-1, increased angiogenesis, and metastatic progression in melanoma. Cancer Detect Prev 1998;22:185–194.
8 Holmgren L, Jackson G, Arbiser J: p53 induces angiogenesis-restricted dormancy in a mouse fibrosarcoma. Oncogene 1998;17:819–824.
9 Hanahan D, Folkman J: Patterns and emerging mechanisms of the angiogenic switch during tumorigenesis. Cell 1996;86:353–364.
10 Mangi MH, Newland AC: Angiogenesis and angiogenic mediators in haematological malignancies. Br J Haematol 2000;111:43–51.
11 Liekens S, De Clercq E, Neyts J: Angiogenesis: Regulators and clinical applications. Biochem Pharmacol 2001;61:253–270.
12 Abedi H, Zachary I: Vascular endothelial growth factor stimulates tyrosine phosphorylation and recruitment to new focal adhesions of focal adhesion kinase and paxillin in endothelial cells. J Biol Chem 1997;272:15442–15451.
13 Mignatti P, Rifkin DB: Plasminogen activators and matrix metalloproteinases in angiogenesis. Enzyme Protein 1996;49:117–137.
14 Suri C, Jones PF, Patan S, Bartunkova S, Maisonpierre PC, Davis S, Sato TN, Yancopoulos GD: Requisite role of angiopoietin-1, a ligand for the TIE2 receptor, during embryonic angiogenesis. Cell 1996;87:1171–1180.
15 Holash J, Wiegand SJ, Yancopoulos GD: New model of tumor angiogenesis: Dynamic balance between vessel regression and growth mediated by angiopoietins and VEGF. Oncogene 1999;18:5356–5362.
16 Breier G, Albrecht U, Sterrer S, Risau W: Expression of vascular endothelial growth factor during embryonic angiogenesis and endothelial cell differentiation. Development 1992; 114:521–532.
17 Singer AJ, Clark RAF: Cutaneous wound healing. N Engl J Med 1999;341:738–746.
18 Mukhopadhyay D, Tsiokas L, Zhou XM, Foster D, Brugge JS, Sukhatme VP: Hypoxic induction of human vascular endothelial growth factor expression through c-Src activation. Nature 1995;375:577–581.
19 Ferrara N, Carver-Moore K, Chen H, Dowd M, Lu L, O'Shea KS, Powell-Braxton L, Hillan KJ, Moore MW: Heterozygous embryonic lethality induced by targeted inactivation of the VEGF gene. Nature 1996;380:439–442.
20 Vincenti V, Cassano C, Rocchi M, Persico G: Assignment of the vascular endothelial growth factor gene to human chromosome 6p21.3. Circulation 1996;93:1493–1495.
21 Tischer E, Mitchell R, Hartman T, Silva M, Gospodarowicz D, Fiddes JC, Abraham JA: The human gene for vascular endothelial growth factor: Multiple protein forms are encoded through alternative exon splicing. J Biol Chem 1991;266:11947–11954.
22 Nicosia RF: What is the role of vascular endothelial growth factor-related molecules in tumor angiogenesis? Am J Pathol 1998;153:11–16.
23 Becker ME: Factors promoting tumor angiogenesis. Cancer Invest 1999;17:594–623.
24 Ferrara N, Alitalo K: Clinical applications of angiogenic growth factors and their inhibitors. Nat Med 1999;5:1359–1364.
25 Brem S: Angiogenesis and cancer control: From concept to therapeutic trial. Cancer Control 1999;6:436–458.
26 Tennant TR, Schaeffer CW, Stadler WM: Angiogenesis inhibitors. Curr Oncol Rep 2000;2: 11–16.
27 Ryan CJ, Wilding G: Angiogenesis inhibitors. New agents in cancer therapy. Drugs Aging 2000;17:249–255.
28 Burrows FJ, Thorpe PE: Vascular targeting – A new approach to the therapy of solid tumors. Pharmacol Ther 1994;64:155–174.
29 Weidner N, Semple JP, Welch WR, Folkman J: Tumor angiogenesis and metastasis – Correlation in invasive breast carcinoma. N Engl J Med 1991;324:1–8.
30 Weidner N, Folkman J, Pozza F, Bevilacqua P, Allred EN, Moore DH, Meli S, Gasparini G: Tumor angiogenesis: A new significant and independent prognostic indicator in early stage breast carcinoma. J Natl Cancer Inst 1992;84: 1875–1887.
31 Macchiarini P, Fontanini G, Hardin MJ, Squartini F, Angeletti CA: Relation of neovascularization to metastasis of non-small-cell lung cancer. Lancet 1992;340:144–146.
32 Weidner N, Carroll PR, Flax J, Blumenfeld W, Folkman J: Tumor angiogenesis correlates with metastasis in invasive prostate carcinoma. Am J Pathol 1993;143:401–409.
33 Vesalainen S, Lipponen P, Talja M, Alhava E, Syrjanen K: Tumor vascularity and basement membrane structure as prognostic factors in T1–2M0 prostatic adenocarcinoma. Anticancer Res 1994;14:709–714.
34 Tanigawa N, Matsumura M, Amaya H, Kitaoka A, Shimomatsuya T, Lu C, Muraoka R, Tanaka T: Tumor vascularity correlates with the prognosis of patients with esophageal squamous cell carcinoma. Cancer 1997;79:220–225.
35 Dickinson AJ, Fox SB, Persad J, Hollyer J, Sibley GN, Harris A: Quantification of angiogenesis as an independent predictor of prognosis in invasive bladder carcinomas. Br J Urol 1994;74:762–766.
36 Jaeger TM, Weidner N, Chew K, Moore DH, Kerschmann RL, Waldman FM, Carroll PR: Tumor angiogenesis correlates with lymph node metastasis in invasive bladder cancer. J Urol 1995;154:69–71.
37 Takahashi Y, Kitadai Y, Bucana CD, Cleary KR, Ellis LM: Expression of vascular endothelial cell growth factor and its receptor, KDR, correlates with vascularity, metastasis, and proliferation of human colon cancer. Cancer Res 1995;55:3964–3968.
38 Tanigawa N, Amaya H, Matsumura M, Shimomatsuya T, Horiuchi T, Muraoka R, Iki M: Extent of tumor vascularization correlates with the prognosis and hematogenous metastasis in gastric carcinomas. Cancer Res 1996;56:2671–2676.
39 Srivastava A, Laidler P, Davies RP, Horgan K, Hughes LE: The prognostic significance of tumor vascularity in intermediate-thickness (0.76–4.0 mm thick) skin melanoma. Am J Pathol 1988;133:419–423.
40 Fox SB, Harris AL: Markers of tumor angiogenesis: Clinical applications in prognosis and anti-angiogenic therapy. Invest New Drugs 1997;15:15–28.
41 DeYoung BR, Wick MR, Fitzgibbon JE, Sirgi KE, Swanson PE: CD31: An immunospecific marker for endothelial differentiation in human neoplasms. Appl Immunohistochem 1993;1:97–100.
42 Van de Rijin M, Rouse RV: CD34: A review. Appl Immunohistochem 1994;2:71–80.
43 Perez-Atayde A, Sallan S, Tedrow U, Connors S, Allred E, Folkman J: Spectrum of tumor angiogenesis in the bone marrow of children with acute lymphoblastic leukemia. Am J Pathol 1997;150:815–821.
44 Aguayo A, Kantarjian H, Manshouri T, Gidel C, Estey E, Thomas D, Koller C, Estrov Z, O'Brien S, Keating M, Freireich E, Albitar M: Angiogenesis in acute and chronic leukemias and myelodysplastic syndromes. Blood 2000; 96:2240–2245.
45 Cao Y, Veitonmaki N, Keough K, Cheng H, Lee LS, Zurakowski D: Elevated levels of urine angiostatin and plasminogen/plasmin in cancer patients. Int J Mol Med 2000;5:547–551.
46 Narendran A, Freedman MH: Pro-angiogenic cytokine pathways in acute lymphoblastic leukemia (abstract 1363). Blood 2000;96(suppl 1):316a.

47 Veiga JP, Sallan SE, Nadler LM, Cardoso AA: Human acute lymphoblastic leukemia promotes angiogenesis in vivo: Pre-clinical models to develop targeted intervention (abstract 484). Blood 2000;96(suppl 1):113a.
48 Padró T, Ruiz S, Bieker R, Bürger H, Steins M, Kienast J, Büchner T, Berdel WE, Mesters RM: Increased angiogenesis in the bone marrow of patients with acute myeloid leukemia. Blood 2000;96:2637–2644.
49 Hussong JW, Rodgers GM, Shami PJ: Evidence of increased angiogenesis in patients with acute myeloid leukemia. Blood 2000;95: 309–313.
50 Di Raimondo F, Palumbo GA, Azzaro MP, Giustolisi R: Angiogenesis in acute myeloid leukemia. Blood 2000;96:3656–3657.
51 Aguayo A, Estey E, Kantarjian H, Mansouri T, Gidel C, Keating M, Giles F, Estrov Z, Barlogie B, Albitar M: Cellular vascular endothelial growth factor is a predictor of outcome in patients with acute myeloid leukemia. Blood 1999;94:3717–3721.
52 Verstovsek S, Estey E, Giles FJ, Manshuri T, Beran M, Rogers A, Keating M, Kantarjian H, Albitar M: Clinical relevance of vascular endothelial growth factor (VEGF) receptors 1 and 2 in acute myeloid leukemia (AML) and myelodysplastic syndromes (MDS) (abstract 441). Blood 2000;94(suppl 1):103a.
53 Lai R, Estey E, Shen Y, Kantarjian H, Gidel C, Beran M, Manshouri T, Quackenbush R, Keating M, Albitar M: Clinical relevance of plasma endostatin levels in patients with acute myeloid leukemia or myelodysplastic syndrome (abstract 455). Blood 2000;96(suppl 1):106a.
54 Pruneri G, Bertolini F, Soligo D, Carboni N, Cortelezzi A, Ferrucci PF, Buffa R, Lambertenghi-Deliliers G, Pezzella F: Angiogenesis in myelodysplastic syndromes. Br J Cancer 1999; 81:1398–1401.
55 Lundberg LG, Lerner R, Sundelin P, Rogers R, Folkman J, Palmblad J: Bone marrow in polycythemia vera, chronic myelocytic leukemia, and myelofibrosis has an increased vascularity. Am J Pathol 2000;157:15–19.
56 Verstovsek S, Kantarjian H, Manshouri T, Keating M, Estey E, Albitar M: Prognostic significance of VEGF protein levels in the bone marrow of patients with chronic myeloid leukemia (abstract 3197). Blood 2000;96(suppl 1):740a.
57 Lunin S, Kantarjian H, Manshouri T, Verstovsek S, Talpaz M, Faderl S, Cortes J, Albitar M: Clinical relevance of Flk1/KDR (VEGF-R2) and (VEGF-R1) proteins in chronic myelogenous leukemia (CML) (abstract 1510). Blood 2000;96(suppl 1):350a.
58 Verstovsek S, Kantarjian H, Manshouri T, Keating M, Estey E, Albitar M: Prognostic significance of Tie-1 protein expression in the bone marrow of patients with chronic myeloid leukemia (abstract 1519). Blood 2000;96(suppl 1):352a.
59 Mesa RA, Hanson CA, Rajkumar SV, Schroeder G, Tefferi A: Evaluation and clinical correlations of bone marrow angiogenesis in myelofibrosis with myeloid metaplasia. Blood 2000; 96:3374–3380.
60 Di Raimondo F, Azzaro MP, Palumbo GA, Bagnato S, Stagno F, Sortino G, Guglielmo P, Giustolisi R: Elevated VEGF serum levels in idiopathic myelofibrosis (abstract 509). Blood 1999;94(suppl 1):116a.
61 Kini AR, Kay NE, Peterson LC: Increased bone marrow angiogenesis in B cell chronic lymphocytic leukemia. Leukemia 2000;14: 1414–1418.
62 Aguayo A, O'Brien S, Keating M, Manshouri T, Gidel C, Barlogie B, Beran M, Koller C, Kantarjian H, Albitar M: Clinical relevance of intracellular vascular endothelial growth factor levels in B-cell chronic lymphocytic leukemia. Blood 2000;96:768–770.
63 Molica S, Vitelli G, Levato D, Gandolfo GM, Liso V: Increased serum levels of vascular endothelial growth factor predict risk of progression in early B-cell chronic lymphocytic leukemia. Br J Haematol 1999;107:605–610.
64 Chen H, Treweeke AT, West DC, Till KJ, Cawley JC, Zuzel M, Toh CH: In vitro and in vivo production of vascular endothelial growth factor by chronic lymphocytic leukemia cells. Blood 2000;96:3181–3187.
65 Duensing S, Atzpodien J: Increased intracellular and plasma levels of basic fibroblast growth factor in B-cell chronic lymphocytic leukemia. Blood 1995;85:1978–1980.
66 Shehata MM, Schwarzmeier JD, Hilgarth M, Hubmann R, Berger R, Lechner K: Implication of transforming growth factor beta in bone marrow fibrosis and myelosuppression in hairy cell leukemia (abstract 1566). Blood 2000; 96(suppl 1):363a.
67 Gruber G, Schwarzmeier JD, Shehata M, Hilgarth M, Berger R: Basic fibroblast growth factor is expressed by CD19/CD11c-positive cells in hairy cell leukemia. Blood 2000;94:1077–1085.
68 Rajkumar SV, Fonseca R, Witzig TE, Gertz MA, Greipp PR: Bone marrow angiogenesis in patients achieving complete response after stem cell transplantation for multiple myeloma. Leukemia 1999;13:469–472.
69 Ribatti D, Vacca A, Nico B, Quondamatteo F, Ria R, Minischetti M, Marzullo A, Herken R, Roncali L, Dammacco F: Bone marrow angiogenesis and mast cell density increase simultaneously with progression of human multiple myeloma. Br J Cancer 1999;79:451–455.
70 Rajkumar SV, Leong T, Roche PC, Fonseca R, Dispenzieri A, Lacy MQ, Lust JA, Witzig TE, Kyle RA, Gertz MA, Greipp PR: Prognostic value of bone marrow angiogenesis in multiple myeloma. Clin Cancer Res 2000;6:3111–3116.
71 Vacca A, Di Loreto M, Ribatti D, Di Stefano R, Gadaleta-Caldarola G, Iodice G, Caloro D, Dammacco F: Bone marrow of patients with active multiple myeloma: Angiogenesis and plasma cell adhesion molecules LFA-1, VLA-4, LAM-1, and CD44. Am J Hematol 1995;50:9–14.
72 Vacca A, Ribatti D, Presta M, Minischetti M, Iurlaro M, Ria R, Albini A, Bussolino F, Dammacco F: Bone marrow neovascularization, plasma cell angiogenic potential, and matrix metalloproteinase-2 secretion parallel progression of multiple myeloma. Blood 1999;93: 3064–3073.
73 Di Raimondo F, Azzaro MP, Palumbo G, Bagnato S, Giustolisi G, Floridia P, Sortino G, Giustolisi R: Angiogenic factors in multiple myeloma: Higher levels in bone marrow than in peripheral blood. Haematologica 2000;85: 800–805.
74 Vacca A, Ribatti D, Ruco L, Giacchetta F, Nico B, Quondamatteo F, Ria R, Iurlaro M, Dammacco F: Angiogenesis extent and macrophage density increase simultaneously with pathological progression in B-cell non-Hodgkin's lymphoma. Br J Cancer 1999;79:965–970.
75 Salven P, Teerenhovi L, Joensuu H: A high pretreatment serum vascular endothelial growth factor concentration is associated with poor outcome in non-Hodgkin's lymphoma. Blood 1997;90:3167–3172.
76 Foss HD, Araujo I, Demel G, Klotzbach H, Hummel M, Stein H: Expression of vascular endothelial growth factor in lymphomas and Castleman's disease. J Pathol 1997;183:44–50.
77 Salven P, Teerenhovi L, Joensuu H: A high pretreatment serum basic-fibroblast growth factor concentration is an independent predictor of poor prognosis in non-Hodgkin's lymphoma. Blood 1999;94:3334–3339.
78 Le Bousse-Kerdilès M-C, Chevillard S, Charpentier A, Romquin N, Clay D, Smadja-Joffe F, Praloran V, Dupriez B, Demory J-L, Jasmin C, Martyré M-C: Differential expression of transforming growth factor-β, basic fibroblast growth factor, and their receptors in CD34+ hematopoietic progenitor cells from patients with myelofibrosis and myeloid metaplasia. Blood 1996;88:4534–4546.
79 Poon RT, Fan S-T, Wong J: Clinical implications of circulating angiogenic factors in cancer patients. J Clin Oncol 2001;19:1207–1225.
80 Nguyen M, Watanabe H, Budson AE, Richie JP, Hayes DF, Folkman J: Elevated levels of an angiogenic peptide, basic fibroblast growth factor, in the urine of patients with a wide spectrum of cancers. J Natl Cancer Inst 1994;86: 356–361.
81 Brunner G, Nguyen H, Gabrilove JL, Rifkin DB, Wilson EL: Basic fibroblast growth factor expression in human bone marrow and peripheral blood cells. Blood 1993;81:631–638.
82 Bikfalvi A, Han ZC: Angiogenic factors are hematopoietic growth factors and vice versa. Leukemia 1994;8:523–529.
83 Bertolini F, Mancusco P, Gobbi A, Pruneri G: The thin red line: Angiogenesis in normal and malignant hematopoiesis. Exp Hematol 2000; 28:993–1000.

84 Wilson EL, Rifkin DB, Kelly F, Hannocks MJ, Gabrilove JL: Basic fibroblast growth factor stimulates myelopoiesis in long-term human bone marrow cultures. Blood 1991;77:954–960.
85 Fajardo LF, Allison AC: Tumor necrosis factor α and angiogenesis; in Bicknell R, Lewis CE, Ferrara N (eds): Tumour Angiogenesis. New York, Oxford University Press, 1997, pp 261–271.
86 Bellamy WT, Richter L, Frutiger Y, Grogan TM: Expression of vascular endothelial growth factor and its receptors in hematopoietic malignancies. Cancer Res 1999;59:728–733.
87 Vacca A, Ribatti D, Iurlaro M, Albini A, Minischetti M, Bussolino F, Pellegrino A, Ria R, Rusnati M, Presta M, Vincenti V, Persico MG, Dammacco F: Human lymphoblastoid cells produce extracellular matrix-degrading enzymes and induce endothelial cell proliferation, migration, morphogenesis, and angiogenesis. Int J Clin Lab Res 1998;28:55–68.
88 Waltenberger J, Claesson-Welsh L, Siegbahn A, Shibuya M, Heldin CH: Different signal transduction properties of KDR and Flt1, two receptors for vascular endothelial growth factor. J Biol Chem 1994;269:26988–26995.
89 Fielder W, Graeven U, Ergun S, Verago S, Kilic N, Stockschlader M, Hossfeld DK: Vascular endothelial growth factor and its receptors in hematopoietic malignancies. Blood 1997;89:1870–1875.
90 Fielder W, Graeven U, Ergun S, Verago S, Kilic N, Stockschlader M, Hossfeld DK: Vascular endothelial growth factor, a possible paracrine growth factor in human acute myeloid leukemia. Am J Pathol 1997;150:1870–1875.
91 Allouche M, Bayard F, Clamens S, Fillola G, Sie P, Almaric F: Expression of basic fibroblast growth factor (b-FGF) and FGF-receptors in human leukemia cells. Leukemia 1995;9:77–86.
92 Konig A, Menzel T, Lynen S, Wrazel L, Rosen A, Al-Katib A, Raveche E, Gabrilove JL: Basic fibroblast growth factor (bFGF) upregulates the expression of bcl-2 in B cell chronic lymphocytic leukemia cell lines resulting in delaying apoptosis. Leukemia 1997;11:258–265.
93 Menzel T, Rahman Z, Calleja E, White K, Wilson EL, Wieder R, Gabrilove J: Elevated intracellular level of basic fibroblast growth factor correlates with stage of chronic lymphocytic leukemia and is associated with resistance to fludarabine. Blood 1996;87:1056–1063.
94 Munshi N, Wilson CS, Penn J, Epstein J, Singhal S, Hough A, Sanderson R, Desikan R, Siegel D, Mehta J, Barlogie B: Angiogenesis in newly diagnosed multiple myeloma: Poor prognosis with increased microvessel density in bone marrow biopsies (abstract). Blood 1998;92(suppl 1):98a.
95 Branemark P-I: Bone marrow microvascular. Structure and Function. Adv Microcirc 1968;1:1–65.
96 Bruyn PPH, Breen PC, Thomas TB: The microcirculation of the bone marrow. Anat Rec 1970;168:55–68.
97 Abboud C, Lichtman M: Structure of the marrow; in Beutler E, Lichtman MA, Coller BS, Kipps TJ (eds): Hematology, ed 5. New York, McGraw-Hill, 1995, p 25.
98 Wagner RC: Endothelial cell embryology and growth. Adv Microcirc 1980;9:45.
99 Andreoni C, Moreau I, Rigal D: Long-term culture of human bone marrow. I. Characterization of adherent cells in flow cytometry. Exp Hematol 1990;18:431–437.
100 Wilkens BS, Jones DB: Vascular networks within the stroma of human long-term bone marrow cultures. Lab Pathol 1995;177:295–301.
101 Shalaby F, Rossant J, Yamaguchi TP, Gertsenstein M, Wu XF, Breitman ML, Schuh AC: Failure of blood-island formation and vasculogenesis in Flk-1-deficient mice. Nature 1995;376:62–66.
102 Sensebe L, Deschaseaux M, Li J, Herve P, Charbord P: The broad spectrum of cytokine gene expression by myoid cells from the human marrow microenvironment. Stem Cells 1997;15:133–143.
103 Thornton DE, Theil K, Payson R, Balcerzak SP, Chiu IM: Characterization of the 5q-breakpoint in an acute nonlymphocytic leukemia patient using pulsed-field gel electrophoresis. Am J Med Genet 1991;41:557–565.
104 Taichman RS, Reilly MJ, Emerson SG: Human osteoblasts support human hematopoietic progenitor cells in in vitro bone marrow cultures. Blood 1996;88:518–524.
105 Veiga JP, Kennan TD, Barata JT, Sallan SE, Nadler LM, Cardoso AA: Peroxisome proliferator-activated receptor-γ (PPAR-γ) expression by bone marrow endothelium reveals a potential target for therapeutic intervention in acute lymphoblastic leukemia (abstract 2785). Blood 1999;94(suppl 1):627a.
106 Veiga JP, Sallan SE, Nadler LM, Cardoso AA: De novo angiogenesis confers a selective advantage to leukemia cells through contact-dependent maintenance of anti-apoptotic gene expression (abstract 2924). Blood 1999;94(suppl 1):658a.
107 Fielder W, Graeven U, Ergun S, Verago S, Kilic N, Stockschlader M, Hossfeld DK: Expression of FLT4 and its ligand VEGF-C in acute myeloid leukemia. Leukemia 1997;11:1234–1237.
108 Brown LF, Detmar M, Tognazzi K, Abu-Jawdeh G, Iruela-Arispe ML: Uterine smooth muscle cells express functional receptors (flt-1 and KDR) for vascular permeability factor/vascular endothelial growth factor. Lab Invest 1997;76:245–255.
109 Yang K, Cepko CL: Flk-1, a receptor for vascular endothelial growth factor (VEGF), is expressed by retinal progenitor cells. J Neurosci 1996;16:6089–6099.
110 Millauer B, Shawver LK, Plate KH, Risau W, Ullrich A: Glioblastoma growth inhibited in vivo by a dominant-negative Flk-1 mutant. Nature 1994;367:576–579.
111 Bredoux C, Uphoff CC, Drexler HG: Expression of tie receptor tyrosine kinase in human leukemia cell lines. Leuk Res 1997;21:595–601.
112 Hashiyama M, Iwama A, Ohshiro K, Kurozumi K, Yasunaga K, Shimizu Y, Masuho Y, Matsuda I, Yamaguchi N, Suda T: Predominant expression of a receptor tyrosine kinase, TIE, in hematopoietic stem cells and B cells. Blood 1996;87:93–101.
113 Batard P, Sansilvestri P, Scheinecker C, Knapp W, Debili N, Vainchenker W, Buhring HJ, Monier MN, Kukk E, Partanen J, Matikainen MT, Alitalo R, Hatzfeld J, Alitalo K: The Tie receptor kinase is expressed by human hematopoietic progenitor cells and by a subset of megakaryocytic cells. Blood 1996;87:2212–2220.
114 Arap W, Pasqualini R, Ruoslahti E: Chemotherapy targeted to tumor vasculature. Curr Opin Oncol 1998;10:560–565.
115 Ruoslahti E: Targeting tumor vasculature with homing peptides from phage display. Semin Cancer Biol 2000;10:435–442.
116 Saiki I, Murata J, Makabe T, Nishi N, Tokura S, Azuma I: Inhibition of tumor angiogenesis by a synthetic cell-adhesive polypeptide containing the Arg-Gly-Asp (RGD) sequence of fibronectin, poly(RGD). Jpn J Cancer Res 1990;81:668–675.
117 Brooks PC, Clark RA, Cheresh DA: Requirement of vascular integrin alpha v beta 3 for angiogenesis. Science 1994;264:569–571.
118 Brooks PC, Montgomery AM, Rosenfeld M, Reisfeld RA, Hu T, Klier G, Cheresh DA: Integrin alpha v beta 3 antagonists promote tumor regression by inducing apoptosis of angiogenic blood vessels. Cell 1994;79:1157–1164.
119 Banks RE, Forbes MA, Kinsey SE, Stanley A, Ingham E, Walters C, Selby PJ: Release of the angiogenic cytokine vascular endothelial growth factor (VEGF) from platelets: Significance for VEGF measurements and cancer biology. Br J Cancer 1998;77:956–964.
120 Aguayo A, Estey E, Kantarjian H, Manshouri T, Rogers A, Giles FJ, Albitar M: Longitudinal analysis of angiogenic factors and vascularity in acute myeloid leukemia (AML) and myelodysplastic syndromes (MDS) (abstract 1380). Blood 2000;96(suppl 1):320a.
121 Flageul B, Wallach D, Cavelier-Balloy B, Bachelez H, Carsuzaa F, Dubertret L: Thalidomide and thrombosis. Ann Dermatol Venereol 2000;127:171–174.
122 Waltham M, Burnand KG, Collins M, Smith A: Vascular endothelial growth factor and basic fibroblast growth factor are found in resolving venous thrombi. J Vasc Surg 2000;32:988–996.
123 Jain RK, Schlenger K, Hockel M, Yuan F: Quantitative angiogenesis assays: Progress and problems. Nat Med 1997;3:1203–1208.
124 O'Reilly MS: The preclinical evaluation of angiogenesis inhibitors. Invest New Drugs 1997;15:5–13.

125 Miller KD, Sweeney CJ, Slegde GW Jr: Redefining the target: Chemotherapeutics as antiangiogenics. J Clin Oncol 2001;19:1195–1206.
126 Clements MK, Jones CB, Cumming M, Daoud SS: Antiangiogenic potential of camptothecin and topotecan. Cancer Chemother Pharmacol 1999;44:411–416.
127 Maragoudakis ME, Peristeris P, Missirlis E, et al: Inhibition of angiogenesis by anthracyclines and titanocene dichloride. Ann NY Acad Sci 1994;732:280–293.
128 Benbow U, Maitra R, Hamilton J, Brinckerhoff CE: Selective modulation of collagenase 1 gene expression by the chemotherapeutic agent doxorubicin. Clin Cancer Res 1999;5:203–208.
129 Paleolog EM, Young S, Stark AC, McCloskey RV, Feldmann M, Maini RN: Modulation of angiogenic vascular endothelial growth factor by tumor necrosis factor alpha and interleukin-1 in rheumatoid arthritis. Arthritis Rheum 1998;41:1258–1265.
130 Presta M, Rusnati M, Belleri M, Morbidelli L, Ziche M, Ribatti D: Purine analogue 6-methylmercaptopurine riboside inhibits early and late phases of the angiogenesis process. Cancer Res 1999;59:2417–2424.
131 Vacca A, Iurlaro M, Ribatti D, Minischetti M, Nico B, Ria R, Pellegrino A, Dammacco F: Antiangiogenesis is produced by nontoxic doses of vinblastine. Blood 1999;94:4143–4155.
132 Kakeji Y, Maehara Y, Ikebe M, Teicher BA: Dynamics of tumor oxygenation, CD31 staining and transforming growth factor-beta levels after treatment with radiation or cyclophosphamide in the rat 13762 mammary carcinoma. Int J Radiat Oncol Biol Phys 1997;37:1115–1123.
133 Browder T, Butterfield CE, Kraling BM, Shi B, Marshall B, O'Reilly MS, Folkman J: Antiangiogenic scheduling of chemotherapy improves efficacy against experimental drug-resistant cancer. Cancer Res 2000;60:1878–1886.
134 Fidler I: Regulation of neoplastic angiogenesis. J Natl Cancer Inst Monogr 2001;51:10–14.
135 Slaton JW, Perrotte P, Inoue K, Dinney CPN, Fidler JJ: Interferon-α-mediated downregulation of angiogenesis-related genes and therapy of bladder cancer are dependent on the optimization of biologic dose and schedule. Clin Cancer Res 1999;5:2726–2734.
136 Quesada JR, Hersh EM, Manning J, Reuben J, Keating M, Schnipper E, Itri L, Gutterman JU: Treatment of hairy cell leukemia with recombinant alpha-interferon. Blood 1986;68:493–497.
137 Di Raimondo F, Fichera E, Pia Azzaro M, Stagno F, Palumob GA, Giustolisi R: Low serum levels of vascular endothelial growth factor (VEGF) and hepatocyte growth factor (HGF) in IFN-treated chronic myeloid leukemia (CML) patients (abstract 4825). Blood 2000;96 (suppl 1):253b.
138 Bhatia R, McCarthy JB, Verfaillie CM: Interferon-α restores normal β-1 integrin-mediated inhibition of hematopoietic progenitor proliferation by the marrow microenvironment in chronic myelogenous leukemia. Blood 1996;88:3883–3891.
139 Sgadari C, Angiolillo AL, Tosato G: Inhibition of angiogenesis by interleukin-12 is mediated by the interferon-inducible protein 10. Blood 1996;88:3877–3882.
140 Voest EE, Kenyon BM, O'Reilly MS, Truitt G, D'Amato RJ, Folkman J: Inhibition of angiogenesis in vivo by interleukin 12. J Natl Cancer Inst 1995;87:581–586.
141 Yao L, Pike SE, Setsuda J, Parekh J, Gupta G, Raffeld M, Jaffe ES, Tosato G: Effective targeting of tumor vasculature by the angiogenesis inhibitors vasostatin and interleukin-12. Blood 2000;96:1900–1905.
142 D'Amato RJ, Loughnan M, Flynn E, Folkman J: Thalidomide is an inhibitor of angiogenesis. Proc Natl Acad Sci USA 1994;91:4082–4085.
143 Kenyon BM, Browne F, D'Amato RJ: Effects of thalidomide and related metabolites in a mouse corneal mode of neovascularization. Exp Eye Res 1997;64:971–978.
144 Sampaio EP, Sarno EN, Galilly R, Chon ZA, Kaplan G: Thalidomide selectively inhibits tumor necrosis factor alpha production by stimulated human monocytes. J Exp Med 1991;173:699–703.
145 Moreira AL, Sampaio EP, Zmuidzinas A, Frindt P, Smith KA, Kaplan G: Thalidomide exerts its inhibitory action on tumor necrosis factor by enhancing mRNA degradation. J Exp Med 1993;177:1675–1680.
146 Turk BE, Jiang H, Liu JO: Binding of thalidomide to 1-acid glycoprotein may be involved in its inhibition of tumor necrosis factor production. Proc Natl Acad Sci USA 1996;93:7552–7556.
147 Singhal S, Mehta J, Desikan R, Ayers D, Roberson P, Eddlemon P, Munshi N, Anaissie E, Wilson C, Dhodapkar M, Zeddis J, Barlogie B: Antitumor activity of thalidomide in refractory multiple myeloma. N Engl J Med 1999;341:1565–1571.
148 Barlogie B: Thalidomide (T) in the management of multiple myeloma (MM): The Arkansas experience in >300 patients (Pts) with single agent (SA) and combination therapy (CT) (abstract 28). Proc Am Soc Clin Oncol 2000;19:9a.
149 Thomas DA: Pilot studies of thalidomide in acute myelogenous leukemia, myelodysplastic syndromes, and myeloproliferative disorders. Semin Hematol 2000;37(suppl 3):26–34.
150 Estey E, Albitar M, Cortes J, Giles F, Thomas D, Koller C, Beran M, Kantarjian H: Addition of thalidomide (T) to chemotherapy did not increase remission rate in poor prognosis AML/MDS (abstract 1394). Blood 2000;96(suppl 1):323a.
151 Thomas DA, Kantarjian HM: Current role of thalidomide in cancer treatment. Curr Opin Oncol 2000;12:564–573.
152 Raza A, Lisak L, Anderews C, Little L, Zorat F, Shetty V, Alvi S, Mundle S, Allampallam K, duRant M, Ekbal M, Muzammil M: Encouraging improvement in cytopenias of patients with myelodysplastic syndromes (MDS) with thalidomide (abstract 111). Proc Am Soc Clin Oncol 2000;19:30a.
153 Mundle S, Zorat F, Shetty V, Allampallam K, Alvi S, Lisak L, Little L, Dean L, Nascimben F, Ekbal M, duRandt M, Broderick E, Venugopal P, Raza A: Biologic determinants of clinical response to thalidomide in myelodysplasia (abstract 626). Blood 2000;96(suppl 1):146a.
154 Vajkoczy P, Menger MD, Vollmar B, Schilling L, Schmiedek P, Hirth KP, Ullrich A, Fong TAT: Inhibition of tumor growth, angiogenesis, and microcirculation by the novel flk-1 inhibitor SU5416 as assessed by intravital multi-fluorescence videomicroscopy. Neoplasia 1999;1:31–41.
155 Fong TAT, Shawver LK, Li S, Tang C, App H, Powell TJ, Kim YH, Schreck R, Wang X, Risau W, Ullrich A, Hirth KP, McMahon G: SU5416 is a potent and selective inhibitor of the vascular endothelial growth factor receptor (Flk1/KDR) that inhibits tyrosine kinase catalysis, tumor vascularization, and growth of multiple tumor types. Cancer Res 1999;59:99–106.
156 Smolich BD, Yuen HA, West KA, Giles FJ, Albitar M, Cherrington JM: The antiangiogenic protein kinase inhibitors SU5416 and SU6668 inhibit the SCF receptor (c-kit) in a human myeloid leukemia cell line and in acute myeloid leukemia blasts. Blood 2001;97:1413–1421.
157 Rosen L, Mulay M, Mayers A, Kabbinavar F, Rosen P, Cropp G, Hannah A: Phase I dose-escalating trial of SU5416, a novel angiogenesis inhibitor in patients with advanced malignancies (abstract 619). Proc Am Soc Clin Oncol 1999;18:161a.
158 Fiedler WM, Tinnefeld H, Mende T, Gehling U, Vohwinkel G, Kelsey S, Scigalla P, Hossfeld DK: A phase II study with SU5416 in patients with C-kit positive AML (abstract 1148). Proc Am Soc Clin Oncol 2001;20:288a.
159 Gordon MS, Talpaz K, Margolin E, Holmgren E, Sledge GW Jr, Benjamin R, Stalter S, Shak S, Adelman D: Phase I trial of recombinant humanized monoclonal anti-vascular endothelial growth factor (anti-VEGF MAB) in patients with metastatic cancer (abstract 1678). Proc Am Soc Clin Oncol 1998;17:210a.
160 Gately S: The contributions of cyclooxygenase-2 to tumor angiogenesis. Cancer Metastasis Rev 2000;19:19–27.
161 Dannhardt G, Kiefer W: Cyclooxygenase inhibitors – Current status and future prospects. Eur J Med Chem 2001;36:109–126.

162 Fosslien E: Molecular pathology of cyclooxygenase-2 in neoplasia. Ann Clin Lab Sci 2000; 30:3–21.
163 Ingber D, Fujita T, Kishimoto S, Sudo K, Kanamaru T, Brem H, Folkman J: Synthetic analogues of fumagillin that inhibit angiogenesis and suppress tumour growth. Nature 1990;348:555–557.
164 Kudelka AP, Levy T, Verschraegen CF, Edwards CL, Piamsomboon S, Termrungruanglert W, Freedman RS, Kaplan AL, Kieback DG, Meyers CA, Jaeckle KA, Loyer E, Steger M, Mante R, Mavligit G, Killian A, Tang RA, Gutterman JU, Kavanagh JJ: A phase I study of TNP-470 administered to patients with advanced squamous cell cancer of the cervix. Clin Cancer Res 1997;3:1501–1505.
165 Kudelka AP, Verschraegen CF, Loyer E: Complete remission of metastatic cervical cancer with the angiogenesis inhibitor TNP-470. N Engl J Med 1998;338:991–992.
166 Dezube BJ, Von Roenn JH, Holden-Wiltse J, Cheung TW, Remick SC, Cooley TP, Moore J, Sommadossi JP, Shriver SL, Suckow CW, Gill PS: Fumagillin analog in the treatment of Kaposi's sarcoma: A phase I AIDS Clinical Trial Group study. AIDS Clinical Trial Group No. 215 Team. J Clin Oncol 1998;16: 1444–1449.
167 Sedlakova O, Sedlak J, Hunakova L, Jakubikova J, Duraj J, Sulikova M, Chovancova J, Chorvath B: Angiogenesis inhibitor TNP-470:Cytotoxic effects on human neoplastic cell lines. Neoplasma 1999;46:283–289.
168 Reuter CWM, Morgan MA, Bergmann L: Targeting the Ras signaling pathway: A rational, mechanism-based treatment for hematologic malignancies. Blood 2000;96:1655–1669.
169 Feldkamp MM, Lau N, Guha A: Growth inhibition of astrocytoma cells by farnesyl transferase inhibitors is mediated by a combination of anti-proliferative, pro-apoptotic and anti-angiogenic effects. Oncogene 1999; 18:7514–7526.
170 Roboz GJ, Dias S, Lam G, Lane WJ, Soignet SL, Warrell RP Jr, Rafii S: Arsenic trioxide induces dose- and time-dependent apoptosis of endothelium and may exert an antileukemic effect via inhibition of angiogenesis. Blood 2000;96:1525–1530.
171 Lew YS, Brown SL, Griffin RJ, Song CW, Kim JH: Arsenic trioxide causes selective necrosis in solid murine tumors by vascular shutdown. Cancer Res 1999;59:6033–6037.
172 Scappaticci FA, Smith R, Pathak A, Schloss D, Lum B, Cao Y, Johnson F, Engleman EG, Nolan GP: Combination angiostatin and endostatin gene transfer induces synergistic antiangiogenic activity in vitro and antitumor efficacy in leukemia and solid tumors in mice. Mol Ther 2001;3:186–196.
173 Klement G, Baruchel S, Rak J, Man S, Clark K, Hicklin DJ, Bohlen P, Kerbel RS: Continuous low-dose therapy with vinblastine and VEGF receptor-2 antibody induces sustained tumor regression without overt toxicity. J Clin Invest 2000;105:R15–R24.
174 Olson TA, Mohanraj D, Roy S, Ramakrishnan S: Targeting the tumor vasculature: Inhibition of tumor growth by a vascular endothelial growth factor-toxin conjugate. Int J Cancer 1997;73:865–870.
175 Regulier E, Paul S, Marigliano M, Kintz J, Poitevin Y, Ledoux C, Roecklin D, Cauet G, Calenda V, Homann HE: Adenovirus-mediated delivery of antiangiogenic genes as an antitumor approach. Cancer Gene Ther 2001;8:45–54.
176 Feldman AL, Libutti SK: Progress in antiangiogenic gene therapy of cancer. Cancer 2000; 89:1181–1194.

Acta Haematologica

Acta Haematol 2001;106:208–213

Antiangiogenic Therapy in Multiple Myeloma

Patrizia Tosi Sante Tura

Institute of Hematology and Medical Oncology 'Seràgnoli', Bologna University, Bologna, Italy

Key Words

Angiogenesis · Multiple myeloma · Thalidomide · Vascular endothelial growth factor

Abstract

In the recent years, several pieces of evidence have pointed out that disease progression in multiple myeloma (MM) is characterized by an increased bone marrow neovascularization. Targeting the mechanisms that control angiogenesis could thus represent an innovative therapeutic approach to MM. Thalidomide, a glutamic acid derivative with sedative properties, is able to inhibit angiogenesis in murine models; this compound has recently demonstrated to be effective in relapsed/refractory MM, leading to a 30–40% response, coupled with mild systemic toxicity. Inhibition of angiogenesis is probably just one of the mechanisms by which thalidomide exerts its action in MM, as immunomodulation and inhibition of cytokine production by bone marrow stroma could also be involved. At present, several studies are ongoing, aiming at testing thalidomide-based drug combinations, mainly with dexamethasone, but also with conventional chemotherapy; the results that have been obtained so far show a synergistic effect of the drug combinations, with a response rate ranging from 50 to 70% in pretreated patients. There is now growing interest in novel compounds with potential antiangiogenic effects, among them a promising activity both in vitro and in animal models has been displayed by thalidomide analogs, inhibitors of vascular endothelial growth factor receptor-2 and endostatin.

Introduction

Multiple myeloma (MM) is a B cell hematological malignancy characterized by proliferation and accumulation of B lymphocytes and plasma cells, secreting monoclonal immunoglobulin, in the bone marrow and, less frequently, at extramedullary sites. The disease shows a progressive clinical course, usually within 3–5 years from diagnosis. Although novel regimens have been introduced through the years, results obtained with conventional chemotherapy have not significantly improved since the introduction of the melphalan + prednisone combination in the late 1960s [1]. Recently, it has been demonstrated that more intensive chemotherapy with single or double autologous stem cell transplantation is superior to conventional chemotherapy as it warrants longer disease-free and overall survival [2, 3]. Allogeneic stem cell transplantation could further improve patient outcome, but it is applicable to a smaller percentage of patients and it is associated with a higher procedure-related morbidity [4, 5]. It should be also pointed out that the relapse rate after

KARGER

Fax + 41 61 306 12 34
E-Mail karger@karger.ch
www.karger.com

0001–5792/01/1064–0208$17.50/0

Accessible online at:
www.karger.com/journals/aha

Dr.ssa Patrizia Tosi
Istituto di Ematologia e Oncologia Medica 'L. e A. Seràgnoli'
Policlinico S. Orsola, Via Massarenti, 9
I–40138 Bologna (Italy)
Tel. +39 051 390413, Fax +39 051 398973, E-Mail ptosi@med.unibo.it

autologous and even allogeneic stem cell transplantation is unfortunately high, and this raises the issue of whether the MM clone can really be eradicated. Novel therapeutic modalities are thus needed in order to find a cure for MM, and insights could derive from a better knowledge of the mechanisms that control MM cell growth and survival. It has recently been reported that angiogenesis plays a central role in MM progression [6, 7], as active disease is characterized by increased bone marrow neovascularization that is paralleled by increased angiogenetic potential of neoplastic plasma cells, mediated by a secretion of basic fibroblast growth factor and vascular endothelial growth factor (VEGF). Inhibition of angiogenesis could thus be worth exploiting in MM therapy. This review focuses on the compounds showing an antiangiogenic activity that has been tested so far in MM, both in experimental systems and in clinical trials.

Thalidomide

Thalidomide is a glutamic acid derivative that has initially been developed for its sedative properties. After the discovery of its teratogenic potential in the early1960s, its use was abandoned. Later on the drug was used in different settings, including cutaneos lepromatosis [8], AIDS-related aphthous ulcers and wasting syndrome [9, 10], cutaneous lesions of systemic lupus erythematosus [11], and cutaneous and pulmonary sarcoidosis [12]. The interest in the drug has also been renewed by demonstration of its activity in chronic graft versus host disease [13, 14], even though poor tolerance frequently limits drug usage in these patients [15]. Thalidomide has shown a broad spectrum of different effects; modulation of T cell activity has been described, with induction of Th2 response and production of IL-2 and γ-interferon [16]; the compound acts also on bone marrow stromal cells causing inhibition of cytokine production, mainly TNF-α [17] but also IL-6 and IL-12 [18]. Thalidomide possesses a potent antiangiogenic activity in experimental systems [19]; it inhibits microvessel formation in the rat aortic ring assay [20] and it decreases vascular density in granulomatous tissue [21]; these effects are probably mediated by inhibition of bFGF and VEGF activity [19, 22, 23]. As a result of its antiangiogenic properties, thalidomide was used in solid tumors such as recurrent gliomas [24] and hormone refractory prostate cancer [25], and minor responses were observed in 2–30% of the cases; there are at present ongoing clinical trials on Kaposi sarcomas and hematological malignancies such as myelofibrosis and chronic myeloid leukemia. Following the observation of a response in 1/5 heavily pretreated refractory MM patients, a clinical trial was started at the University of Arkansas in 1997 [26]. Eighty-four patients with relapsed refractory MM, most of whom had been previously submitted to autologous stem cell transplantation, were treated with thalidomide at 200 mg/day, increasing the dose by 200 mg every 2 weeks to a maximum of 800 mg/day. A >25% decrease in serum or urine paraprotein was observed in 32% of the patients, with 2 patients achieving a complete remission; median time to response was 1.5 months, median response duration was longer than 14.5 months. Since these data had been reported, several groups have studied the effects of thalidomide in relapsed/refractory MM, obtaining comparable results [27–33] (table 1). Side effects encountered upon thalidomide therapy were mainly sedation, constipation and skin rash; these effects are generally mild, but they can condition patients' quality of life and can lead to discontinuation of therapy, especially when high doses are administered [34]. Furthermore, the occurrence of peripheral neuropathy, though rare, should not be overlooked, due to possible permanent effects [35]. Toxic epidermal necrolysis and pulmonary embolism have also been reported in few patients as anecdotal events [36, 37]. It has not been clarified yet if there is a dose-response effect of thalidomide therapy, so that what the optimal drug dosage should be is still a matter of debate. Barlogie et al. [38], updating the results of the Arkansas trial, demonstrated that the cumulative dose at 3 months represents a predictor of response; conversely other groups [27, 39] have shown that responses can be achieved at doses as low as 200 mg/day and even at 50 mg/day [40]. After wide testing in relapsed/refractory patients, there are at present ongoing trials, using thalidomide, either alone or in combination, as first-line thera-

Table 1. Single agent thalidomide in relapsed/refractory MM

Authors	Ref. No.	Patients	Thalidomide dose/day	Response %
Singhal et al., 1999	26	84	200→800	32
Weber et al., 1999	27	46	200→800	50
Juliusson et al., 2000	29	23	200→800	43
Kneller et al., 2000	28	17	200→800	64
Hideshima et al., 2000	32	44	200→800	39
Yakoub-Agha et al., 2000	31	83	200→800	66
Pini et al., 2000	30	5	200	70
Tosi et al., 2001	33	11	200→800	72

Table 2. Thalidomide + dexamethasone combinations

Authors	Ref. No.	Patients status	Thalidomide dose/day	Dexamethasone dose/schedule	Response %
Weber et al., 2000	45	47/relapsed/ refractory	200→800	20 mg/m²/day days 1–5, 15–18	52 (>50%)
Dimopoulos et al., 2000	46	38/relapsed/ refractory	200→400	40 mg/m²/day days 1–4, 9–12, 17–20 then days 1–4/month	52 (>50%)
Rajikumar et al., 2000	41	26 untreated	200→800	40 mg/m²/day days 1–4, 9–12, 17–20 odd courses days 1–4/even courses	77 (>50%)
Palumbo et al., 2000	47	37/relapsed/ refractory	100	40 mg/m² days 1–4/month	75 (>25%)

py in MM. Rajikumar et al. [41] have shown a 38% response rate in untreated patients with smouldering MM; this is comparable to what is obtained in pretreated patients. Although these results are preliminary, they support the concept that thalidomide exerts its antineoplastic activity through pathways that are different from those followed by conventional antineoplastic therapy. Whether bone marrow angiogenesis is really perturbed by thalidomide therapy, however, is still under investigation. Early observations by Singhal et al. [26] showed no difference in bone marrow microvessel density comparing bone marrow biopsies of sensitive and resistant patients. Conversely, Cheng et al. [42] demonstrated that an increased pretreatment microvessel density could predict the response to therapy. VEGF secretion by MM cell lines is not influenced by in vitro treatment with thalidomide according to Rajikumar et al. [43], while Weber et al. [44] demonstrated that VEGF serum levels were higher in responding patients. Given these contrasting results, although inhibition of bone marrow angiogenesis has been claimed to be the major mechanism of thalidomide action in MM, other mechanisms could also be involved, such as immunomodulation and inhibition of cytokine production by bone marrow stroma. Indirect evidence supporting the cooperation of multiple pathways in thalidomide activity could be represented by the relative rapid response (1–2 months) in sensitive patients.

Thalidomide-Based Drug Combinations

Aiming at improving the results obtained with thalidomide as a single agent, several groups have tested the compound in combination with drugs that are known to be active in MM. Most clinical trials have been designed adding dexamethasone to thalidomide [41, 45–47] (table 2); the combination improved the efficacy of thalidomide and was also effective in patients who had previously turned out to be resistant to thalidomide or dexamethasone alone [46]. In newly diagnosed patients, oral thalidomide + dexamethasone determined a 77% response, which is comparable, or even superior, to what can be obtained with VAD infusional chemotherapy. Other studies were conducted using thalidomide in combination with conventional chemotherapy; Moehler et al. [48] evaluated thalidomide plus cyclophosphamide-etoposide-dexamethasone (CED) in poor-prognosis MM patients, obtaining 7% complete responses and 71% partial responses; Kropff et al. [49] used hyperfractionated cyclophosphamide in combination with thalidomide in relapsed/refractory MM patients, achieving 86% partial response; Munshi et al. [50] combined thalidomide with cyclophosphamide, etoposide, doxorubicin, cisplatin and dexamethasone (DT PACE) in patients with aggressive MM or plasma cell leukemia; 40% response was obtained with no adverse effects on subsequent stem cell collection.

Thalidomide Analogs

The pleiotropic effects shown by thalidomide prompted investigators to find compounds with more selective activity, in order to better understand the mechanism of action of thalidomide and to drugs that could potentially target the disease with fewer side effects. Two classes of thalidomide analogs have been synthesized so far; they include phosphodiesterase-4 inhibitors that inhibit

TNF-α production but have no effects on T cells (selected cytokine inhibitory drugs), and phosphodiesterase-4 inhibitors that stimulate T cell activation and IL-2 and γ-interferon production (immunomodulatory drugs) [32]. These latter seem more promising as they have shown superior activity in reducing DNA synthesis and in inducing apoptosis in MM cell lines and in bone marrow plasma cells from MM patients.

Endostatin

Endostatin is a terminal fragment of collagen that inhibits endothelial cell proliferation [51]. In the SCID-hu host system this compound has been demonstrated to inhibit MM growth and tumor burden, reflected by a reduction in serum levels of human monoclonal immunoglobulins. Furthermore, mice bone density was preserved, as demonstrated by X-ray evaluation [52].

VEGF Inhibitors

VEGF is a potent angiogenic protein that acts directly on endothelial cells, promoting cell growth and survival [53]. Three high affinity VEGF receptors have been identified on endothelial cells; VEGFR-2 (Flk/KDR) has been recognized to be the major receptor transducing the effects of VEGF. Activation of VEGFR-2 stimulates release of tissue factor, proliferation, chemotaxis and sprouting of endothelial cells in vitro and enhances angiogenesis in vivo [54]. VEGF has been demonstrated to be produced by neoplastic plasma cells [55] and increased VEGF levels have been found in sera obtained from peripheral blood and bone marrow of MM patients [56]. Bone marrow stromal cells from MM patients possess VEGFR-2; stimulation with VEGF results in IL-6 release, leading to the hypothesis that VEGFR-2 inhibition could in turn reduce MM growth in vivo [55, 57]. At present, several VEGFR-2 inhibitors have been tested in vitro and in vivo in animal models; some of these compounds are undergoing phase I–II clinical trial in solid tumors such as colon and prostate cancer [58] and Kaposi sarcoma; they include ribozymes that target VEGFR mRNA, anti-VEGFR monoclonal antibodies and small molecules that act as catalytic inhibitor of VEGFR-2 protein kinase by binding the adenine pocket of the intracellular moiety. These latter compounds seem the most promising in MM [59].

Conclusions

Despite the introduction of high dose (sub)myeloablative regimens, the therapy of MM is far from being fully satisfactory, especially in terms of long-lasting remission. In the attempt at finding a cure for the disease, newer treatment modalities should be exploited. As neovascularization is a process related to full-blown disease, targeting angiogenesis could be a therapeutic approach worth pursuing. Thalidomide, a potent inhibitor of angiogenesis, has recently been recognized as the third most effective weapon in MM treatment, together with alkylating agents and corticosteroids. Inhibition of angiogenesis is probably just one of the mechanisms by which thalidomide exerts its action, as immunomodulation and inhibition of cytokine production can also be involved; however, the striking efficacy of thalidomide, both alone and in combination with other anti-MM compounds, makes it worthwhile using it more widely in this disease. Other potentially useful drugs, such as thalidomide analogs, endostatin and VEGF inhibitors are undergoing in vitro and in vivo testing, and will soon be available for clinical use. For the future, however, further studies are needed in order to achieve a better understanding of the biology of MM; this will help design drugs with a more selective activity against the mechanisms of myelomagenesis that will hopefully help to improve the outcome of this disease.

Acknowledgements

This work was supported in part by MURST (S.T.).

References

1 Gregory WM, Richards MA, Malpas JS: Combination chemotherapy versus melphalan and prednisolone in the treatment of multiple myeloma: An overview of published trials. J Clin Oncol 1992;10:334–342.

2 Attal M, Harousseau JL, Stoppa AM, Sotto JJ, Fuzibet JG, Rossi JF, Casassus P, Maisonneuve H, Facon T, Ifrah N, Payen C, Bataille R: A prospective, randomized trial of autologous bone marrow transplantation and chemotherapy in multiple myeloma. N Engl J Med 1996;335:91–97.

3 Barlogie B, Jagannath S, Vesole DH, Nancke S, Cheson B, Mattox S, Bracy D, Salmon S, Jacobson J, Crowley J, Tricot G: Superiority of tandem autologous transplantation over standard therapy for previously untreated multiple myeloma. Blood 1997;98:789–793.

4 Gahrton G, Tura S, Ljungman P, Belanger C, Brandt L, Cavo M, Facon T, Granena A, Gore M, Gratwohl A: Allogeneic bone marrow transplantation in multiple myeloma. European Group for Bone Marrow Transplantation. N Engl J Med 1991;325:1267–1273.

5 Cavo M, Bandini G, Benni M Gozzetti A, Ronconi S, Rosti GA, Zamagni E, Lemoli RM, Bonini A, Belardinelli A, Motta MR, Rizzi S, Tura S: High-dose busulfan and cyclophosphamide are an effective conditioning regimen for allogeneic bone marrow transplantation in chemosensitive multiple myeloma. Bone Marrow Transplant 1998;22:27–32.

6 Vacca A, Ribatti D, Presta M, Minischetti M, Iurlaro M, Ria R, Albini A, Bussolino F, Dammacco F: Bone marrow neovascularization, plasma cell angiogenic potential, and matrix metalloproteinase-2 secretion parallel progression of human multiple myeloma. Blood 1999; 93:3064–3073.

7 Vacca A, Ribatti D, Iurlaro M, Albini A, Minischetti M, Bussolino F, Pellegrino A, Ria R, Rusnati M, Presta M, Vincenti V, Persico MG, Dammacco F: Human lymphoblastoid cells produce extracellular matrix-degrading enzymes and induce endothelial cell proliferation, migration, morphogenesis, and angiogenesis. Int J Clin Lab Res 1998;28:55–68.

8 Shannon EJ, Ejigu M, Haile Mariam HS, Berhan TY, Tasesse G: Thalidomide's effectiveness in erythema nodosum leprosum is associated with a decrease in CD4+ cells in the peripheral blood. Lepr Rev 1992;63:5–11.

9 Jacobson JM, Spritzler J, Fox L, Fahey JL, Jackson JB, Chernoff M, Wohl DA, Wu AW, Hooton TM, Sha BE, Shikuma CM, MacPhail LA, Simpson DM, Trapnell CB, Basgoz N: Thalidomide for the treatment of esophageal aphthous ulcers in patients with human immunodeficiency virus infection. J Infect Dis 1999; 180:61–67.

10 Reyes Teran G, Sierra Madero JG, Martinez del Cerro V, Arroyo Figueroa H, Pasquetti A, Calva JJ, Ruiz Palacios GM: Effects of thalidomide on HIV-associated wasting syndrome: A randomized, placebo-controlled clinical trial. AIDS 1996;10:1501–1507.

11 Stevens RJ, Andujar C, Edwards CJ, Ames PR, Barwick AR, Khamashta MA, Hughes GR: Thalidomide in the treatment of cutaneous manifestations of lupus erythematosus: Experience in sixteen consecutive patients. Br J Rheumatol 1997;36:353–359.

12 Carlesimo M, Giustini S, Rosi A, Bonaccorsi P, Calvieri S: Treatment of cutaneous and pulmonary sarcoidosis with thalidomide. J Am Acad Dermatol 1995;32:866–869.

13 Heney D, Norfolk DR, Wheeldon J, Bailey CC, Lewis IJ, Barnard DL: Thalidomide treatment for chronic graft-versus-host disease. Br J Haematol 1991;78:23–27.

14 Vogelsang GB, Farmer ER, Hess AD, Altamonte V, Beschorner WE, Jabs DA, Corio RL, Levin LS, Colvin OM, Wingard JR: Thalidomide for the treatment of chronic graft-versus-host disease. N Engl J Med 1992;326:1055–1058.

15 Parker PM, Chao N, Nademanee A, O'Donnell MR, Schmidt GM, Snyder DS, Stein AS, Smith EP, Molina A, Stepan DE: Thalidomide as salvage therapy for chronic graft-versus-host disease. Blood 1995;86:3604–3609.

16 Haslett PA, Corral LG, Albert M, Kaplan G: Thalidomide costimulates primary human T lymphocytes, preferentially inducing proliferation, cytokine production, and cytotoxic responses in the CD8+ subset. J Exp Med 1998; 187:1885–1892.

17 Sampaio EP, Sarno EN, Galilly R, Cohn ZA, Kaplan G: Thalidomide selectively inhibits tumor necrosis factor production by stimulated human monocytes. J Exp Med 1991;173:699–703.

18 Moller DR, Wysocka M, Greenlee BM, Ma X, Wahl L, Flockhart DA, Trinchieri G, Karp CL: Inhibition of IL-12 production by thalidomide. J Immunol 1997;159:5157–5161.

19 Folkmann J: What is the evidence that tumors are angiogenesis dependent. J Natl Cancer Inst 1990;82:4–6.

20 Bauer KS, Dixon SC, Figg WD: Inhibition of angiogenesis by thalidomide requires metabolic activation, which is species-dependent. Biochem Pharmacol 1998;55:1827–1834.

21 Or R, Feferman R, Shoshan S: Thalidomide reduces vascular density in granulation tissue of subcutaneously implanted polyvinyl alcohol sponges in guinea pigs. Exp Hematol 1998;26: 217–221.

22 D'Amato RJ, Loughnan MS, Flynn E, Folkmann J: Thalidomide is an inhibitor of angiogenesis. Proc Natl Acad Sci USA 1994;91: 4082–4085.

23 Kenyon BM, Browne F, D'Amato RJ: Effects of thalidomide and related metabolites in a mouse corneal model of neovascularization. Exp Eye Res 1997;64:971–978.

24 Fine HA, Figg WD, Jaekle K, Wen PY, Kyritsis AP, Loeffler JS, Levin VA, Black PM, Kaplan R, Pluda JM, Yung WK: Phase II trial of the antiangiogenic agent thalidomide in patients with recurrent high grade gliomas. J Clin Oncol 2000;18:708–715.

25 Figg WD, Raje S, Bauer KS, Tompkins A, Venzon D, Bergan R, Chen A, Hamilton M, Pluda J, Reed E: Pharmacokinetics of thalidomide in an elderly prostate cancer population. J Pharmacol Sci 1999;88:121–125.

26 Singhal S, Metha J, Desikan R, Ayers D, Robertson P, Eddlemon P, Munshi N, Anaissie E, Wilson C, Dhodapkar M, Zeldis J, Barlogie B: Antitumor activity of thalidomide in refractory multiple myeloma. N Engl J Med 1999;341: 1565–1571.

27 Weber DM, Gavino M, Delasalle K, Rankin K, Giralt S, Alexanian R: Thalidomide alone or with dexamethasone for multiple myeloma. Blood 1999;94(suppl 1):604a.

28 Kneller A, Raanani P, Hardan I, Avigdor A, Levi I, Berkowicz M, Ben-Bassat I: Therapy with thalidomide in refractory multiple myeloma patients – The revival of an old drug. Br J Haematol 2000;108:391–393.

29 Juliusson G, Celsing F, Turesson I, Lenhoff S, Adriansson M, Malm C: Frequent good partial remissions from thalidomide including best response ever in patients with advanced refractory and relapsed myeloma. Br J Haematol 2000; 109:89–96.

30 Pini M, Baraldi A, Pietrasanta D, Allione B, Depaoli L, Salvi F, Levis A: Low-dose thalidomide in the treatment of refractory myeloma. Haematologica 2000;85:1111–1112.

31 Yakoub-Agha I, Attal M, Dumontet C, Moreau P, Berthou C, Lamy T, Grosbios B, Dauriac C, Dorvaux I, Bay JO, Monconduit M, Harousseau JL, Duguet C: Thalidomide in patients with advanced myeloma: Survival and prognostic factors. Blood 2000;96(suppl 1):167a.

32 Hideshima T, Chauhan D, Shima Y, Raje N, Davies FE, Tai YT, Treon SP, Lin B, Schlossman RL, Richardson P, Muller G, Stirling DI, Anderson KC: Thalidomide and its analogs overcome drug resistance of human multiple myeloma cells to conventional chemotherapy. Blood 2000;96:2943–2950.

33 Tosi P, Ronconi S, Zamagni E, Cellini C, Grafone T, Cangini D, Pileri SA, Tura S, Baccarani M, Cavo M: Salvage therapy with thalidomide in multiple myeloma patients relapsing after autologous peripheral blood stem cell transplantation. Haematologica 2001;86:409–413.

34 Rodrigues J, Oyama Y, Burt R, Traynor A: Achievement of minimal disease response to thalidomide is limited by patient tolerance more often than disease resistance. Blood 2000; 96(suppl 1):294b.

35 Calabrese L, Fleischer AB: Thalidomide: Current and potential clinical applications. Am J Med 2000;108:487–495.

36 Rajikumar SV, Gertz MA, Witzig TE: Life-threatening toxic epidermal necrolysis with thalidomide therapy for myeloma. N Engl J Med 2000;343:972–973.

37 Zangari M, Anaissie E, Desikan R, Badros A, Morris C, Munshi N, Gopal AV, Fink L, Spoon D, Tricot G, Barlogie B: Thalidomide-induced hypercoagulability in multiple myeloma (MM). Blood 2000;96(suppl 1):296b.

38 Barlogie B, Spencer T, Tricot G, Zeldis J, Munshi N, Zangari M, Badros A, Toor A, Shaughnessy J: Long-term follow-up of 169 patients receiving a phase II trial of single agent thalidomide for advanced and refractory multiple myeloma (MM). Blood 2000;96(suppl 1):514a.
39 Larkin M: Low-dose thalidomide seems to be effective in multiple myeloma. Lancet 1999; 354:925.
40 Durie BGM, Stepan DE: Efficacy of low-dose thalidomide (T) in multiple myeloma. Blood 1999;94(suppl 1):316a.
41 Rajikumar SV, Hayman S, Fonseca R, Dispenzieri A, Lacy MQ, Geyer S, Wellik L, Lust JA, Kyle RA, Greipp PR, Gertz MA, Witzig TE: Thalidomide plus dexamethasone (thal/dex) and thalidomide alone (thal) as first line therapy for newly diagnosed multiple myeloma. Blood 2000;96:168a.
42 Cheng D, Kini AR, Rodriguez J, Burt R, Peterson LC, Traynor AE: Microvascular density and cytotoxic T cell activation correlate with response to thalidomide in multiple myeloma patients. Blood 1999;94(suppl 1):317a.
43 Rajikumar SV, Timm M, Mesa RA, Fonseca R, Dispenzieri A, Lacy MQ, Lust JA, Gertz MA, Kyle RA, Greipp PR, Witzig TE: Effect of thalidomide on myeloma cell apoptosis and VEGF secretion. Blood 2000;96(suppl 1):364a.
44 Weber DM, Rankin K, Gavino M, Delasalle K, Aguayo A, Albitar M, Alexanian R: Angiogenesis factors and sensitivity to thalidomide in previously untreated multiple myeloma. Blood 2000;96(suppl 1):168a.
45 Weber DM, Rankin K, Gavino M, Delasalle K, Alexanian R: Thalidomide + dexamethasone for resistant multiple myeloma. Blood 2000; 96(suppl 1):167a.
46 Dimopoulos MA, Zervas K, Galani E, Grigoraki V, Vervessou E, Samantas E, Kiamouris C, Gika D, Papadimitriou C, Anagnostopoulos N: Thalidomide and dexamethasone combination for multiple myeloma refractory to dexamethasone-based regimens. Blood 2000;96:286b.
47 Palumbo A, Giaccone L, Bertola A, Bringhen S, Rus C, Triolo S, Pileri A, Boccadoro M: Thalidomide and dexamethasone as salvage therapy for refractory and relapsed myeloma. Blood 2000;96:292b.
48 Moehler TM, Neben K, Hawighorst H, Egerer G, van Kaick G, Ho AD, Goldschmidt H: Thalidomide plus ced chemotherapy as salvage therapy in poor prognosis multiple myeloma. Blood 2000;96(suppl 1):290b.
49 Kropff MH, Innig G, Mitterer M, Straka C, Ostermann H, Kock OM, Berdel WE, Kienast J: Hyperfractionated cyclophosphamide in combination with pulsed dexamethasone and thalidomide (hyper-CTD) in primary refractory or relapsed multiple myeloma. Blood 2000; 96(suppl 1):168a.
50 Munshi N, Desikan R, Zangari M Badros A, Chodimella U, Toor A, Cromer J, Terry J, Anaissie E, Barlogie B: Chemoangiotherapy with dt-pace for previously treated myeloma. Blood 1999;94(suppl 1):123a.
51 O'Rielly MS, Boehm T, Shing Y, Fukai N, Vasios G, Lane WS, Flynn E, Birkhead JR, Olsen BR, Folkman J: Endostatin: An endogenous inhibitor of angiogenesis and tumor growth. Cell 1997;88:277–285.
52 Fujii R, Yaccoby S, Epstein J: Control of myeloma growth with the anti-angiogenic agent endostatin. Blood 2000;96(suppl 1):360a.
53 Ferrara N, Davis-Smyth T: The biology of vascular endothelial growth factor. Endocr Rev 1997;18:4–25.
54 Karkkainen MJ, Petrova TV: Vascular endothelial growth factor receptors in the regulation of angiogenesis and lymphangiogenesis. Oncogene 2000;19:5598–5605.
55 Bellamy WT, Richter L, Frutiger Y, Grogan TM: Expression of vascular endothelial growth factor and its receptors in hematopoietic malignancies. Cancer Res 1999;59:728–733.
56 Di Raimondo F, Azzaro MP, Palumbo GA, Bagnato S, Giustolisi G, Floridia PM, Sortino G, Giustolisi R: Angiogenic factors in multiple myeloma: Higher levels in bone marrow than in peripheral blood. Haematologica 2000;85: 800–805.
57 Dankbar B, Padrò T, Leo R, Feldmann B, Kropff M, Mesters RM, Serve H, Berdel WE, Kienast J: Vascular endothelial growth factor and interleukin-6 in paracrine tumor-stromal interactions in multiple myeloma. Blood 2000; 95:2630–2636.
58 Gordon MS, Margolin K, Talpaz M, Sledge GW, Holmgren E, Benjamin R, Stalter S, Shak S, Adelman DC: Phase I safety and pharmacokinetic study of recombinant human antivascular endothelial growth factor in patients with advanced cancer. J Clin Oncol 2001;19:843–850.
59 Anderson KC, Kyle RA, Dalton WS, Landowski T, Shain K, Jove R, Hazelhurst L, Berenson J: Multiple myeloma: New insights and therapeutic approaches. Hematology 2000;72:147–165.

Acta Haematologica

Acta Haematol 2001;106:214–219

Angiogenesis and Hereditary Hemorrhagic Telangiectasia

Rendu-Osler-Weber Disease

Carlo Sabbà[a] Anna Cirulli[a] Rita Rizzi[b] Giovanna Pasculli[a]
Mauro Gallitelli[a] Giorgina Specchia[b] Vincenzo Liso[b]

[a]Cattedra di Medicina d'Urgenza e Pronto Soccorso, and [b]Cattedra di Ematologia, Università degli Studi, Bari, Italy

Key Words
Angiogenesis · Rendu-Osler-Weber disease · Telangiectasia

Abstract
To date much of the recent work on pathological angiogenesis has focused on inflammatory diseases, diabetes and cancer in particular. Hereditary hemorrhagic telangiectasia or Rendu-Osler-Weber disease provides an example of the genetic disorder of angiogenesis in which a multisystemic angiodysplasia is responsible for severe hemorrhage. The disease pathogenesis is partially explained by a defect in the TGF-β signaling system, although in more recent works a possible role of other vascular growth factors has been proposed. This paper provides a model of an aberrant angiogenesis in which multiple vascular growth factors could be involved in a diffuse angiodysplasia.

Introduction

In the last decade a diffuse interest in the understanding of the complex cascade of events leading to blood vessel formation has been growing. Several studies have focused on the second phase of this process, the angiogenesis, during which the primitive capillary plexus, through both pruning and vessel enlargement, forms the interconnecting branching pattern characteristic of the mature vasculature [1]. In addition to its role during development, angiogenesis also occurs in the organism in postnatal life; it is necessary in physiological processes like wound healing and reproductive functions, as well as in a variety of disorders including tumor growth and metastasis, rheumatoid arthritis, and retinopathies [2].

The possibility of stimulating new vessels formation in ischemic heart disease or peripheral arteriopathy or to cure cancer or inflammatory disorders by suppressing excessive vessel growth represents an intriguing prospective [3, 4]. A less known disease, characterized by an aberrant angiogenesis whose pathogenetic pathway has so far not been clarified, is hereditary hemorrhagic telangiectasia (HHT). This is an autosomal dominant genetic disorder characterized by hemorrhage and vascular malformations (mucocutaneus telangiectases and visceral arteriovenous malformations, AVMs) due to a diffuse angiodysplasia [5].

KARGER
Fax + 41 61 306 12 34
E-Mail karger@karger.ch
www.karger.com

0001–5792/01/1064–0214$17.50/0

Accessible online at:
www.karger.com/journals/aha

Prof. Vincenzo Liso
Unità Operativa di Ematologia, Università degli Studi di Bari
Piazza Giulio Cesare, 11
I–70124 Bari (Italy)
Tel. +39 080 559 23 37, Fax +39 080 542 89 78, E-Mail ematba@cimedoc.uniba.it

Pathogenesis of HHT: A Genetic Disorder of Angiogenesis

In HHT angiodysplastic lesions affect many organs such as brain, lung, liver, gastrointestinal tract, skin and nose and are responsible for severe and recurrent bleedings [5]. The involvement of visceral vascular beds seems to increase with age and a significant variation in clinical expression is seen between patients and even among members of the same family [6]. Mutations occur in two genes encoding for vascular endothelial transmembrane proteins: endoglin on chromosome 9 and ALK-1 (activin receptor-like kinase 1) on chromosome 12 [7, 8] and at least a third unknown locus has been predicted [9]. Endoglin and ALK-1 represent type III and type I TGF-β receptor [7, 8] and identify, respectively, two different types of HHT: HHT type 1, more frequently characterized by pulmonary AVM, and HHT type 2. The TGF-β superfamily includes several cytokines which modulate the synthesis of extracellular matrix, endothelial cell migration, proliferation and differentiation [10].

It has been hypothesized that the involvement of TGF-β in the HHT pathogenesis leads to a perturbation of vascular development and homeostasis [11]; several studies have been performed in order to elucidate the exact mechanism by which endoglin and ALK-1, interacting with TGF-β, induce a diffuse angiodysplasia.

Endoglin

Endoglin is a homodimeric transmembrane glycoprotein primarily expressed on vascular endothelial cells so that it is recognized as an endothelial cell marker (CD-105). It is also present on activated monocytes, syncytiotrophoblasts, pre-B lymphoid leukemic cells [12] and is upregulated on vascular endothelial cells in tumors [13], psoriasis and in response to UV irradiation [14, 15]. Endoglin represents type III of TGF-β receptors. It binds TGF-β1 and TGF-β3 with high affinity through type II TGF-β receptor and modulates the transduction of TGF-β signaling [16]. The exact role of endoglin in TGF-β signaling and in HHT pathogenesis is still unclear but recent studies may lead to new hypotheses. At least 29 different mutations of the endoglin gene have been identified [17].

Pece et al. [18] showed, in cultured cells, that mutant endoglin is rarely present in HHT type 1 patients and only half of the normal copies of endoglin is expressed at the cell surface. This suggests that haploinsufficiency is responsible for HHT. More recently, the generation of animal models of HHT provides a better way of investigating the endoglin role in vasculogenesis and angiogenesis. Li et al. [19] observed that mice lacking endoglin died at gestational day 11.5 and that they showed poor vascular smooth muscle development and stopped endothelial remodelling. Furthermore, in contrast to mice lacking TGF-β1, vasculogenesis defects were not described. Mice lacking one ($Eng^{+/-}$) or both ($Eng^{-/-}$) copies of the gene have been generated. $Eng^{-/-}$ embryos died of a defective heart and vascular development by gestational day 10–10.5. Endoglin was found to be normally present on the endothelium of knockout embryos, yolk sack and placenta until gestational day 9.0. Thus, in situ differentiation of precursors (angioblasts) to endothelial cells, their assembling in the vascular labyrinth of the yolk sack, placenta and embryos and the generation of native vessels connected to the primitive heart do not need endoglin. On the other hand, some $Eng^{+/-}$ mice exhibited signs of HHT, such as recurrent epistaxis and telangiectases; some others developed normally.

In summary, endoglin does not seem to be required for the early phase of vasculogenesis; it plays an important role in the growth and remodelling of the primitive capillary network into a complex network through proliferation and migration of endothelial cells. In addition, endoglin appears to be essential for heart valve formation and septation [20]. The presence of HHT clinical manifestations only in some of the mice with a certain genetic background and the variety of clinical settings among these animals prompt that the involvement of other modified genes or epigenetic factors, such as shear stress or hormonal levels, may explain the heterogeneity of the disease. This even represents a common aspect of the human disease, in which particular vascular malformations develop only in genetically predisposed individuals and clinical manifestations vary between members of the same family having an identical endoglin mutation [21]. Thus HHT is thought to be a genetically and clinically heterogeneous disorder.

ALK-1

ALK-1 is a type 1 receptor of the TGF-β superfamily and is expressed on vascular endothelial cells. To date seven types of TGF-β1 receptor (ALK-1 to 7) and, in a patient with HHT type 2, at least 17 different kinds of mutations in ALK-1 have been identified.

Several studies demonstrated that ALK-1 interacts with growth factor/receptor complexes composed of either TGF-β1/TGF-β type II receptor or activin/activin type II receptor though no downstream signaling occurs [22–24]. TGF-β1 and TGF-β3, as well as a third unknown ligand present in the serum, can activate chimeric ALK-1 [25]. However, since ALK-1 does not elicit a specific transcriptional response [26, 27] it was considered an 'orphan' receptor.

An overexpression of ALK-1 was found in human lung and placenta [22, 23]. Lung expression increase in the early postnatal period may be the result of an increase in the pulmonary vasculature [28]. A murine model provided evidence of a high distribution of ALK-1 at gestational day 8 at sites of vasculogenesis in both embryonic and extraembryonic tissues, in giant trophoblast cells and in decidua blood vessel endothelia. At days 9–12 ALK-1 was highest in blood vessels, lung mesenchyme and at sites of epithelial mesenchymal interaction [29]. This pattern of expression of ALK-1 is very similar to that of TGF-β1 [30] suggesting a potential role in vascular development.

In order to elucidate the function of ALK-1 during blood vessel formation, Oh et al. [31] inactivated the ALK-1 gene in mice by gene targeting. Heterozygous mice (ALK-$1^{+/-}$) were normal, therefore ALK-1 mutation did not have a dominant effect. Knockout mice died at midgestation showing an excessive fusion of capillary plexus into cavernous vessels and hyperdilation of large vessels. In addition, this work demonstrated that the vascular defects were associated with an increased expression of angiogenic factors and proteases and were distinguished by defective differentiation and recruitment of smooth muscle cells. In other words, mice lacking ALK-1 exhibit blood vessel defects similar to those observed in mice lacking TGF-β1, TGF-β type II receptor or endoglin confirming that ALK-1 may mediate TGF-β1 signal in endothelial cells.

Endoglin and ALK-1 in TGF-β Signaling

It is well known that the TGF-β superfamily includes several cytokines, such as TGF-βs, activins, bone morphogenetic proteins and others, which regulate many aspects of cellular proliferation, differentiation, adhesion, migration and extracellular matrix formation. TGF-β is thought to play an important role in the vascular remodelling and in the maintenance of vessel wall integrity: it modulates the activities of other angiogenic factors in endothelial cell proliferation and migration, production or degradation of extracellular matrix, interaction of endothelial and smooth muscle cells in the process of physiological and pathological angiogenesis [10].

Activated by the contact between endothelial and mesenchymal cells, TGF-β1 induces differentiation of mesenchymal cells into pericytes and smooth muscle cells, stabilizing the endothelial tube [32]. TGF-β1 or TGF-β type II receptor null mice die at 10.5 gestational day showing a primary defect in yolk sack vasculogenesis and hematopoiesis [33]. TGF-β3 knockout mice die soon after birth exhibiting pleural hemorrhage and fragile and dilated pulmonary capillaries and veins [34, 35]. This led to the assumption that there may be a possible role of TGF-β1 and TGF-β3 in the development of lung vasculature and the impairment of their usual function might contribute to the pathology of pulmonary AVMs [36]. There is still a long way to go to fully understand the exact role of endoglin and ALK-1 in TGF-β1 signaling, and therefore in HHT pathogenesis.

The transmission of TGF-β signals from the cell surface to the nucleus requires a complex of receptors and cytosolic Smad proteins. Endoglin and ALK-1 are, respectively, type III and type I TGF-β receptors. Endoglin accelerates the binding of TGF-β to the type II TGF-β receptor on endothelial cells; subsequently type II TGF-β receptor phosphorylates type I TGF-β receptor, ALK-5 and ALK-1, and phosphorylated ALK-5 and ALK-1 activate the downstream proteins Smad 2/3 and Smad 1/5, respectively. These Smads dissociate from the type I TGF-β receptor, bind to Smad 4 and, entering the nucleus, regulate transcription from specific gene promoters involved in angiogenesis [37].

Several studies demonstrated that TGF-β has a biphasic effect on angiogenesis dependent on its concentration [38]. This suggests that the endothelial response to TGF-β may also be concentration-dependent. A biphasic effect may be justified by the use of two different receptors, TGF-βR-1 and ALK-1, with different affinities for TGF-β. Furthermore endoglin has been hypothesized to be required as a receptor partner for both type 1 receptors in order to maintain the balance between positive and negative regulation of angiogenesis. This pattern is complicated by the identification of a novel ligand, which could play a part in ALK-1 antagonistic activity at different time points. Alternatively in ALK-1 signaling this unknown ligand might elicit other angiogenic responses, TGF-β independently [39].

Vascular abnormalities in ALK-1 knockout mice may depend on the persistence of the activation phase of angiogenesis, during which the endothelial cells degrade the perivascular basement membrane, invade the extracellular space, proliferate and form capillary lumen. Furthermore, ALK-1 seems to regulate the transition of the endothelial cells from the activation to the resolution phase of angiogenesis, characterized by the cessation of endothelial cell proliferation and restitution of the basement membrane. In addition a balance model for the role of TGF-β1 signaling in angiogenesis is proposed in endothelial cells (ECs). The TGF-β signal is mediated by two signaling pathways, ALK-1 and ALK-5, in ECs. Activation of ALK-1 leads to the EC resolution phase where angiogenic factors and proteinases, such as vascular endothelial growth factor (VEGF) and plasminogen activator, are repressed; the TGF-β1 signal mediated by ALK-5 transforms ECs into the activation phase, where angiogenic factors and proteinases are suppressed. In HHT type 1 endoglin mutation damages both the ALK-1 and ALK-5 pathways, whereas only the ALK-1 pathway is disrupted in HHT type 2, leading to the dominance of the ALK-5 signaling one. This stimulates the activation phase of ECs and results in arteriovenous connections between dilated venules and arteries.

The most intriguing question is: how can gene abnormalities of endoglin and ALK-1 result in an identical phenotype in a dominant inherited pattern [37]? In this regard a more complex pattern is suggested: endoglin appears to activate TGF-β1 signaling by both facilitating the formation and becoming part of the type II receptor. Thus a reduced dosage of endoglin, in HHT type 1 patients, may give a significant decrease in TGF-β1 concentration, impairing the ALK-1 and ALK-5 pathways. Therefore, having a higher sensitivity to TGF-β1 than ALK-1, the ALK-5 pathway remains unaffected and induces arteriovenous connections between dilated venules and arterioles with no intervening capillary bed [40]. On the other hand, high concentrations of TGF-β1 activate the ALK-1 pathway, which inhibits the ALK-5 and leads to the resolution phase of angiogenesis. This may explain both the biphasic effect of TGF-β1 on ECs and the expression of identical phenotypes in mutations of two different genes such as endoglin and ALK-1.

VEGF in HHT

In a recent paper HHT is described interestingly as an excellent example of blood vessel growth and enlargement providing a model to study this second phase in angiogenesis [41]. An analysis of 500 HHT patients provided evidence of a significant reduction in the incidence of atherosclerosis and coronary artery disease as compared to the general population [Guttmacher, pers. commun.]. Jacobson [41] hypothesizes that the incidence could be the same, but HHT patients were asymptomatic because of their great ability to form collateral arteries in the heart. The analysis of the cellular aspects of the telangiectases and the larger AVMs in various tissues of patients could provide important elements to better understand the various steps leading to vascular malformations. Unfortunately few works on this have been reported. The analysis of the ultrastructure of dermal telangiectases of different sizes revealed that the earliest alterations in the vasculature of HHT are focally dilated postcapillary venules. Then, these venules increase in size, develop disproportionate layers of smooth muscle cells and connect through capillaries to dilated arterioles. The last step consists of further enlargement to about 2 mm and loss of capillaries. A perivascular leukocytic infiltrate composed mostly of lymphocytes is seen around the arteriovenous connection but not around the normal vasculature of affected patients [42]. Similar analyses, performed on the large visceral AVMs, have so far not been reported. However, it has been hypothesized that factors acting at a local level in different tissues may be implicated in the genesis of vascular malformations so heterogeneous in size, although the pathogenetic mechanism should be the same [41].

The identification of two distinct genes, endoglin and AKL-1, and the analysis of their functions in the TGF-β1 signaling pathway only partially explain the complete cascade of events leading to the aberrant blood vessel formations in HHT.

Endoglin is found to be equally expressed both in cerebral AVMs (CAVMs) and pulmonary AVMs (PAVMs) as well as in normal blood vessels, suggesting that all blood vessels in HHT type 1 patients express reduced endoglin in situ and that AVMs are not attributed to a focal loss of endoglin. Thus it has been hypothesized that other factors and/or receptors might be involved in CAVMs and PAVMs formation. Both VEGF and angiopoietin 1 receptor (Tie-2 receptor) were found overexpressed in the endothelium of CAVMs [43, 44]; moreover, angiopoietin and Tie-2 are implicated in the regulation of the interaction between endothelial and mesenchymal cells and their matrix [45–47]. This appears to be consistent with a possible role of VEGF, Ang 1 and Tie-2 in HHT vascular malformations [48, 20].

On the other hand, as regards VEGF, it is possible that its increased expression in AVMs may be dependent on the impaired balance between ALK-1 and ALK-5 pathways, as proposed in Oh's model. In other words the expression of VEGF may be an effect of the aberrant angiogenic signal and not one of the causal factors.

In order to evaluate whether VEGF is increased at serum levels in HHT patients as compared to normal subjects and whether it could be considered a marker of the disease, we investigated a serum level of this growth factor in a group of HHT patients (pers. commun.). Our preliminary data have shown higher values of serum VEGF in HHT patients relative to healthy subjects, even if the difference between the two groups did not reach a statistical significance. Further analyses, in larger groups of patients, are needed in order to elucidate whether serum VEGF could eventually represent a useful marker of HHT for screening.

Other factors, besides VEGF and Ang 1, have been hypothesized to be involved in triggering and/or propagating the formation of vascular malformations in HHT.

An immune response arising from perivascular leukocytes at the site of the telangiectases or from the smooth muscle cells could play a part in this scenario. These adjunctive steps in the formation of telangiectases may take place during pre- and postnatal development and may compensate for or overcome the haploinsufficiency of the reduced production of endoglin. This is consistent with the differences of expression of HHT lesions in individuals even within the same family and with the observation that incomplete gene penetrance might not be so rare in HHT [41].

In summary, it is likely that, since a multitude of growth factors are involved in normal angiogenesis, the aberrant blood vessel formation in HHT results from a perturbation of physiological effects of these growth factors in vascular development and homeostasis. In addition other gene mutations and epigenetic factors such as shear stress and environmental conditions could be implicated in the generation of vascular malformations.

References

1 Risau W: Mechanism of angiogenesis. Nature 1997;386:671–674.
2 Folkman J: Angiogenesis in cancer, vascular rheumatoid and other disease. Nat Med 1995; 1:27–31.
3 Folkman J: Clinical applications of research on angiogenesis. N Engl J Med 1995;333:1757–1763.
4 Pepper MS: Positive and negative regulation of angiogenesis: From cell biology to the clinic. Vasc Med 1997;1:253–266.
5 Guttmacher AE, Marchuk DA, White RI Jr: Hereditary hemorrhagic telangiectasia. N Engl J Med 1995;333:918–924.
6 Plauchu H, de Chadarevian JP, Bideau A, Robert JM: Age-related clinical profile of hereditary hemorrhagic telangiectasia in an epidemiologically recruited population. Am J Med Genet 1989;32:291–297.
7 McAllister KA, Grogg KM, Johnson DW, Gallione CJ, Baldwin MA, Jackson CE, Helmbold EA, Markel DS, McKinnon WC, Murrell J: Endoglin, a TGF-beta binding protein of endothelial cells, is the gene for hereditary haemorrhagic telangiectasia type 1. Nat Genet 1994;8: 345–351.
8 Johnson DW, Berg JN, Baldwin MA, Gallione CJ, Marondel I, Yoon SJ, Stenzel TT, Speer M, Pericak-Vance MA, Diamond A, Guttmacher AE, Jackson CE, Attisano L, Kucherlapati R, Porteous ME, Marchuk DA: Mutations in the activin receptor-like kinase 1 gene in hereditary haemorrhagic telangiectasia type 2. Nat Genet 1996;13:189–195.
9 Piantanida M, Buscarini E, Dellavecchia C, Minelli A, Rossi A, Buscarini L, Danesino C: Hereditary haemorrhagic telangiectasia with extensive liver involvement is not caused by either HHT1 or HHT2. J Med Genet 1996;33: 441–443.
10 Pepper MS: Transforming growth factor-beta: Vasculogenesis, angiogenesis, and vessel wall integrity. Cytokine Growth Factor Rev 1997;8: 21–43.
11 Shovlin CL, Scott J: Inherited diseases of the vasculature. Annu Rev Physiol 1996;58:483–507.
12 Bellon T, Corbi A, Lastres P, Cales C, Cebrian M, Vera S, Cheifetz S, Massague J, Letarte M, Bernabeu C: Identification and expression of two forms of the human transforming growth factor-beta-binding protein endoglin with distinct cytoplasmic regions. Eur J Immunol 1993;23:2340–2345.
13 Thorpe PE, Burrows FJ: Antibody-directed targeting of the vasculature of solid tumors. Breast Cancer Res Treat 1995;36:237–251.
14 Wang JM, Kumar S, van Agthoven A, Kumar P, Pye D, Hunter RD: Irradiation induces up-regulation of E9 protein (CD105) in human vascular endothelial cells. Int J Cancer 1995; 62:791–796.
15 Wang JM, Kumar S, Pye D, van Agthoven AJ, Krupinski J, Hunter RD: A monoclonal antibody detects heterogeneity in vascular endothelium of tumours and normal tissues. Int J Cancer 1993;54:363–370.
16 Barbara NP, Wrana JL, Letarte M: Endoglin is an accessor protein that interacts with the signaling receptor complex of multiple members of transforming growth factor-β superfamily. J Biol Chem 1999;274:584–594.
17 Marchuk DA: Genetic abnormalities in hereditary hemorrhagic telangiectasia. Curr Opin Hematol 1998;5:332–338.
18 Pece N, Vera S, Cymerman U, White RI Jr, Wrana JL, Letarte M: Mutant endoglin in hereditary hemorrhagic telangiectasia type 1 is transiently expressed intracellularly and is not a dominant negative. J Clin Invest 1997;100: 2568–2579.
19 Li DY, Sorensen LK, Brooke BS, Urness LD, Davis EC, Taylor DG, Boak BB, Wendel DP: Defective angiogenesis in mice lacking endoglin. Science 1999;284:1534–1537.
20 Bourdeau A, Dumont DJ, Letarte M: A murine model of hereditary hemorrhagic telangiectasia. J Clin Invest 1999;104:1343–1351.
21 Shovlin CL, Hughes JM, Scott J, Seidman CE, Seidman JG: Characterization of endoglin and identification of novel mutations in hereditary hemorrhagic telangiectasia. Am J Hum Genet 1997;61:68–79.
22 Attisano L, Carcamo J, Ventura F, Weis FM, Massague J, Wrana JL: Identification of human activin and TGF beta type I receptors that form heteromeric kinase complexes with type II receptors. Cell 1993;75:671–680.
23 ten Dijke P, Ichijo H, Franzen P, Schulz P, Saras J, Toyoshima H, Heldin CH, Miyazono K: Activin receptor-like kinases: A novel subclass of cell-surface receptors with predicted serine/threonine kinase activity. Oncogene 1994;8:2879–2887.

24 Ryden M, Imamura T, Jornval H, Belluardo N, Nevue I, Trupp M, Okadome T, ten Dijke P, Ibanez CF: A novel type I receptor serine-threonine kinase predominantly expressed in the adult central nervous system. J Biol Chem 1996;271:30603–30609.
25 Lux A, Attisano L, Marchuk DA: Assignment of transforming growth factor beta1 and beta3 and a third new ligand to the type I receptor ALK-1. J Biol Chem 1999;274:9984–9992.
26 Kretzschmar M, Massagué J: SMADs: Mediators and regulators of TGF-beta signaling. Curr Opin Genet Dev 1998;8:103–111.
27 Bassing CH, Yingling JM, Howe DJ, Wang T, He WW, Gustafson ML, Shah P, Donahoe PK, Wang XF: A transforming growth factor beta type I receptor that signals to activate gene expression. Science 1994;263:87–89.
28 Panchenko MP, Williams MC, Brody JS, Yu Q: Type I receptor serine-threonine kinase preferentially expressed in pulmonary blood vessels. Am J Physiol 1996;270:L547–L558.
29 Roelen B, van Rooijen M, Mummery CL: Expression of ALK-1, a type 1 serine/threonine kinase receptor, coincides with sites of vasculogenesis and angiogenesis in early mouse development. Dev Dyn 1997;209:418–430.
30 Dickson K, Philip A, Warshawsky H, O'Connor-McCourt M, Bergeron JJ: Specific binding of endocrine transforming growth factor-beta 1 to vascular endothelium. J Clin Invest 1995;95:2539–2554.
31 Oh SP, Seki T, Goss KA, Imamura T, Yi Y, Donahoe PK, Li L, Miyazono K, ten Dijke P, Kim S, Li E: Activin receptor-like kinase 1 modulates transforming growth factor-beta 1 signaling in the regulation of angiogenesis. Proc Natl Acad Sci USA 2000;97:2626–2631.
32 Folkman J, D'Amore PA: Blood vessel formation: What is its molecular basis? Cell 1996;87:1153–1155.
33 Dickson MC, Martin JS, Cousins FM, Kulkarni AB, Karlsson S, Akhurst RJ: Defective haematopoiesis and vasculogenesis in transforming growth factor-beta 1 knockout mice. Development 1995;121:1845–1854.
34 Proetzel G, Pawlowski SA, Wiles MV, Yin M, Boivin GP, Howles PN, Ding J, Ferguson MW, Doetschman T: Transforming growth factor-beta 3 is required for secondary palate fusion. Nat Genet 1995;11:409–414.
35 Kaartinen V, Voncken JW, Shuler C, Warburton D, Bu D, Heisterkamp N, Groffen J: Abnormal lung development and cleft palate in mice lacking TGF-beta 3 indicates defects of epithelial-mesenchymal interaction. Nat Genet 1995;11:415–421.
36 Shovlin C, Letarte M: Hereditary hemorrhagic telangiectasia and pulmonary arteriovenous malformations: Issues in clinical management and review of pathogenic mechanisms. Thorax 1999;54:714–729.
37 Azuma H: Genetic and molecular pathogenesis of hereditary hemorrhagic telangiectasia. J Med Invest 2000;47:81–90.
38 Pepper MS, Vassalli JD, Orci L, Montesano R: Biphasic effect of transforming growth factor-beta 1 on in vitro angiogenesis. Exp Cell Res 1993;204:356–363.
39 Lux A, Attisano L, Marchuk DA: Assignment of transforming growth factor beta1 and beta3 and a third new ligand to the type I receptor ALK-1. J Biol Chem 1999;274:9984–9992.
40 Carmeliet P, Schoonjans L, Kieckens L, Ream B, Degen J, Bronson R, De Vos R, van den Oord JJ, Collen D, Mulligan RC: Physiological consequences of loss of plasminogen activator gene function in mice. Nature 1994;368:419–424.
41 Jacobson BS: Hereditary hemorrhagic telangiectasia: A model for blood vessel growth and enlargement. Am J Pathol 2000;156:737–742.
42 Braverman IM, Keh A, Jacobson BS: Ultrastructure and three-dimensional organization of the telangiectases of hereditary hemorrhagic telangiectasia. J Invest Dermatol 1990;95:422–427.
43 Sonstein WJ, Kader A, Michelsen WJ, Llena JF, Hirano A, Casper D: Expression of vascular endothelial growth factor in pediatric and adult cerebral arteriovenous malformations: An immunocytochemical study. J Neurosurg 1996;85:838–845.
44 Hatva E, Jaaskelainen J, Hirvonen H, Alitalo K, Haltia M: Tie endothelial cell-specific receptor tyrosine kinase is upregulated in the vasculature of arteriovenous malformations. J Neuropathol Exp Neurol 1996;55:1124–1133.
45 Puri MC, Rossant J, Alitalo K, Bernstein A, Partanen J: The receptor tyrosine kinase TIE is required for integrity and survival of vascular endothelial cells. EMBO J 1995;14:5884–5891.
46 Suri C, Jones PF, Patan S, Bartunkova S, Maisonpierre PC, Davis S, Sato TN, Yancopoulos GD: Requisite role of angiopoietin-1, a ligand for the TIE2 receptor, during embryonic angiogenesis. Cell 1996;87:1171–1180.
47 Sato TN, Tozawa Y, Deutsch U, Wolburg-Buchholz K, Fujiwara Y, Gendron-Maguire M, Gridley T, Wolburg H, Risau W, Qin Y: Distinct roles of the receptor tyrosine kinases Tie-1 and Tie-2 in blood vessel formation. Nature 1995;376:70–74.
48 Bourdeau A, Cymerman U, Paquet ME, Meschino W, McKinnon WC, Guttmacher AE, Becker L, Letarte M: Endoglin expression is reduced in normal vessels but still detectable in arteriovenous malformations of patients with hereditary hemorrhagic telangiectasia type 1. Am J Pathol 2000;156:911–923.

Acta Hæmatologica

Author Index Vol. 106, No. 4, 2001

Subject Index Vol. 106, No. 4, 2001

KARGER

Fax + 41 61 306 12 34
E-Mail karger@karger.ch
www.karger.com

Accessible online at:
www.karger.com/journals/aha

Acta Hæmatologica

Author Index Vol. 106, 2001

KARGER
Fax + 41 61 306 12 34
E-Mail karger@karger.ch
www.karger.com

Accessible online at:
www.karger.com/journals/aha

Subject Index Vol. 106, 2001

Acta Hæmatologica

KARGER
Fax + 41 61 306 12 34
E-Mail karger@karger.ch
www.karger.com

Accessible online at:
www.karger.com/journals/aha

Vol. 106, 2001

Affiliated with Molecular Biology of Hematopoiesis Symposium

Acta Hæmatologica

Founded 1948 by E. Meulengracht, K. Rohr, and G. Rosenow
Continued by H. Lüdin (1960–1977), U. Bucher (1977–1983), R.S. Hillman (1978–1987), H.R. Marti (1983–1988), E.A. Beck (1984–1988), B. Ramot (1989–1995)

KARGER

Basel · Freiburg · Paris · London · New York ·
New Delhi · Bangkok · Singapore · Tokyo · Sydney

S. Karger
Medical and Scientific Publishers
Basel · Freiburg · Paris · London
New York · New Delhi · Bangkok
Singapore · Tokyo · Sydney

Drug Dosage
The authors and the publisher have exerted every effort to ensure that drug selection and dosage set forth in this text are in accord with current recommendations and practice at the time of publication. However, in view of ongoing research, changes in government regulations, and the constant flow of information relating to drug therapy and drug reactions, the reader is urged to check the package insert for each drug for any change in indications and dosage and for added warnings and precautions. This is particularly important when the recommended agent is a new and/or infrequently employed drug.

Printed in Switzerland on acid-free paper by
Reinhardt Druck, Basel

KARGER

Fax + 41 61 306 12 34
E-Mail karger@karger.ch
www.karger.com

Contents Vol. 106, 2001

Acta Haematologica

No. 1–2

No. 3

KARGER

Fax + 41 61 306 12 34
E-Mail karger@karger.ch
www.karger.com

Access to full text and tables of contents, including tentative ones for forthcoming issues:
www.karger.com/journals/aha/aha_bk.htm

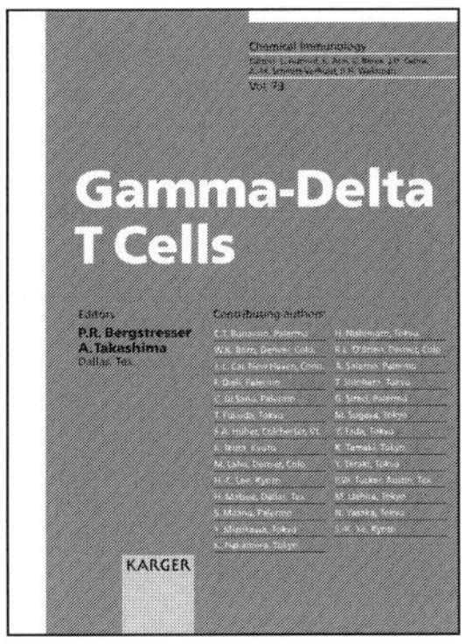

Gamma-Delta T Cells
KARGER

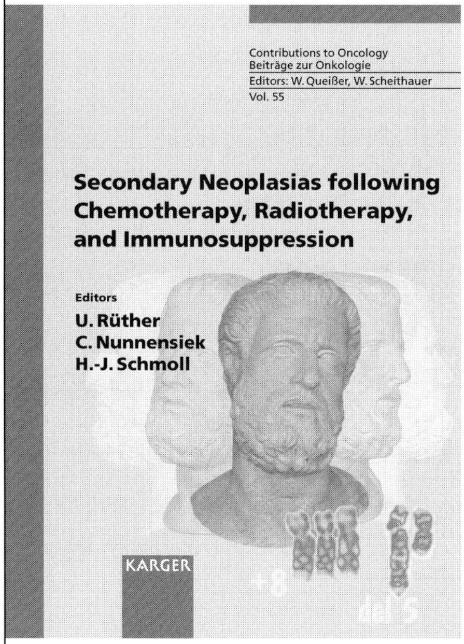

Secondary Neoplasias following Chemotherapy, Radiotherapy, and Immunosuppression

Editors

U. Rüther
C. Nunnensiek
H.-J. Schmoll

Oncology; Transplantation, Radiology

Complete remissions and survival times of tumor patients are increasing steadily – and so is the risk of developing therapy-associated secondary malignancy. At the same time, we face the growing diagnostic and therapeutic problem of tumorigenesis during posttransplantation immunosuppressive therapy.

The *theoretical section* delves into the various causes of tumorigenesis, with special chapters on secondary chemo- and/or radiotherapy-induced tumorigenesis and neoplasia occurring during posttransplantation immunosuppressive therapy. The risk of individual cytostatic agents causing secondary malignoma is covered, as are the functions and dysfunctions of immunosurveillance. The immune system's methods of recognizing tumors are also examined, and specific information on the role of herpesviruses in organ transplantation is included. The *clinical part* of the book portrays in depth major hematologic and oncologic malignancies that can arise after chemo- and/or radiotherapy administered after organ transplantation.

With this book, clinical hemato-oncologists and those working in transplantation will gain greater insight into the risks, genesis and complications of secondary malignancy – but also into its treatment today and in the future. Last but most certainly not least, the importance of international collaboration for the advancement of diagnosis and therapy is underscored – as is reflected by the international team of contributing authors.

KI 01225

Contents

www.karger.com/bookseries/coonc

Contributions to Oncology / Beiträge zur Onkologie, Vol. 55
Series Editors: Queißer, W. (Mannheim); Scheithauer, W. (Wien)
ISSN 0250–3220

Secondary Neoplasias following Chemotherapy, Radiotherapy, and Immunosuppression
Editors: Rüther, U. (Ludwigsburg); Nunnensiek, C. (Reutlingen); Schmoll, H.-J. (Halle/Saale)
VIII + 376 p., 38 fig., 8 in color, 22 tab., hard cover, 2000
CHF 198.– / DEM 257.– / USD 172.25
Prices subject to change
DEM price for Germany, USD price for USA only
ISBN 3–8055–7116–X

KARGER

Order Form

Please send: ____ copy/ies

Postage and handling free with prepayment

Payment:
☐ Check enclosed ☐ Please bill me

Please charge to my credit card
☐ American Express ☐ Diners ☐ Eurocard
☐ MasterCard ☐ Visa

Card No.: ____________

Exp. date: ____________

Orders may be placed with any bookshop, subscription agency, directly with the publisher or through a Karger distributor.

Fax: +41 61 306 12 34
S. Karger AG, P.O. Box, CH–4009 Basel (Switzerland)
E-Mail karger@karger.ch, **www.karger.com**

Name/Address: ____________

____

____

____

____

Date: ____________

Signature: ____________